Person-Centred Approaches to Dementia Care

Person-Centred Approaches to Dementia Care

Ian Morton

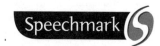

Speechmark Publishing Ltd
Telford Road • Bicester • Oxon OX26 4LQ • UK

To my Mum and Dad

About the Author

Ian Morton graduated with a degree in Philosophy in 1978 and after training to become a nurse in Mental Health, has been working with people with dementia since 1985. He spent five years as a charge nurse on the Felix Post Unit at the Maudsley Hospital, before becoming manager of Beauvale Court Day Centre in Nottingham, which serves those with dementia who remain in their own homes. In addition he has worked as Dementia Care Mapping Project Co-ordinator for the Nottingham Healthcare Trust, and has written several articles on both Validation Therapy and Dementia Care.

Published by
Speechmark Publishing Ltd, Telford Road, Bicester, Oxon OX26 4LQ, UK
www.speechmark.net

Reprinted 2002

002-3115/Printed in the United Kingdom/1010

British Library Cataloguing in Publication Data

Morton, Ian, 1957–
   Person-centred approaches to dementia care. – (Winslow editions)
   1. Dementia – Patients – Care   2. Client-centred psychotherapy
   I. Title
   362.1'9683
ISBN 0 86388 423 7
(Previously published by Winslow Press Ltd under ISBN 0 86388 227 7)

Contents

Figures

Tables

Acknowledgements

W HILE WRITING A BOOK can often feel like the loneliest occupation on earth it is, as perceptive authors have noted before, a much more collaborative venture than it might appear. In a book such as this, which largely reviews the work of others, the co-operation of those whose work is being discussed is essential and in this regard I remain indebted to, Janet Bell, Naomi Feil, Fiona Goudie, Tom Kitwood, Vicki de Klerk-Rubin and Iain McGregor for agreeing to share with me some of their time and thoughts. Whilst Graham Stokes (in view of a potential conflict of interest!) was kept away from this process, his patience and support as commissioning editor was as valuable as his insightful comments on the earlier drafts of the text.

Dion van Werde, whom I have yet to meet in person, demonstrated how a combination of telephone, e-mail and fax can overcome the barrier of the North Sea and form the basis of a productive and enjoyable relationship. Those innovative ideas which appear in our joint chapter were entirely the results of Dion's work and expertise, and if I have acted as a simple gateway through which Pre-Therapy passes into the world of dementia care I will be more than satisfied. The advice, comments and guidance offered by Cate Simmons were instrumental in the production of Chapter 1 and I have her to thank for any understanding I possess as to what 'person-centred' *really* means.

Looking back on a longer term basis, I must mark the supportive influence of Christine Bleathman without whom the potential reward of working with people with dementia would have passed me by many years ago. Other helpful colleagues from my time working on the Felix Post Unit at the Maudsley Hospital are too numerous to name, but I cannot fail to mention Chris Hart (not least because he mentioned me) whose 'affirmation therapy' remains, even after this work, a mysteriously neglected contribution to the field. More recently, colleagues — particularly Lynn Powdrill and Ann Palmer — from Beauvale Court Day Centre deserve my thanks, as do those who have come to visit us each week over the past six years. I have counted myself as fortunate to work within the Health Care of the Elderly Directorate of Nottingham Healthcare Trust, and especially with Pat Anderson, Sheila Gibson and Doreen Shepherd.

The greatest heroes were, as ever, on the home front, and to Annie, Billy and Sally I owe a thousand thanks, and almost as many weekends.

Tom Kitwood

This book would never have been written were it not for the work of Tom Kitwood. I say this not simply because his writings form such a large part of the subject matter, but rather because the appearance of a person-centred agenda in British dementia care is primarily a result of his influence. The full extent of that influence became clear when I learnt, with a shock and dismay shared by so many, of his sudden death shortly before this book went to press. Over the following days I became increasingly conscious of the enormous gap that is left now that he is no longer with us. It is a gap, a silence, that we shall be aware of for a long time to come.

CHAPTER 1

The Origins of Person-Centred Care

The Beginnings of a Person-Centred Tradition in Dementia Care?

Hindsight tempts us to view the arrival and development of a 'person-centred' approach to dementia care as having been almost inevitable. We might, borrowing a concept from the economists, suggest that the laws of supply and demand made it so.

On the demand side, we can cite the explosion of the demographic 'time bomb' — a marked growth in that section of the population in which the incidence of dementia increases significantly. While estimates vary, a consensus of studies claim that Britain alone will be home to between 750,000 and one million people with dementia during the first decade of the twenty-first century, heightening public concern over an approaching 'epidemic' at a time when the prospects for developing a significant pharmacological response remain remote.

Such circumstances give rise to an understandable insistence that a proper degree of attention be paid to the quality of care provided for people who develop dementia, with psychological care being at the forefront of concern. The encouraging burst of energy and creativity that has characterised the development of care practice in recent years cannot overshadow the fact that carers, paid and unpaid alike, continue to suffer from a collective lack of preparation for their role. With some noteworthy exceptions, systematic research into the area of care, as opposed to cure, remains sadly neglected.

If this accounts, in some part, for an increase in the demand for new and better approaches to dementia care then the person-centred tradition was always likely to form part of the supply. The roots of this tradition are to be found in the theory and practice of the 'client-centred' psychotherapy pioneered by the American psychologist Carl Rogers in the years that followed the Second World War. Since the early 1960s the influence of the ideas underpinning his approach has spread far beyond the individual psychotherapy which spawned them, leaving their mark on many aspects of culture and thought throughout the western world. In 1975 Rogers' biographer, Richard Evans, was able to claim that:

> Professionals from education, religion, nursing, medicine, psychiatry, law, business, government, public health, law enforcement, race relations, social work — the list goes on and on — all came to feel that here, finally, was an approach which enabled them to succeed in the previously neglected human dimensions of their jobs.
> (Evans, 1975)

The earliest published evidence of Rogerian influence gaining a foothold in the field of dementia care is found in an article by Naomi Feil, published in 1967. Some 20 years were to pass, however, before this influence was to take root in Britain. The strands of this process which form the central subjects of this book — Feil's Validation Therapy, the development of Resolution Therapy, the work of Tom Kitwood and the Bradford Dementia Group — have been accompanied by an abundance of conferences, workshops and articles advocating the adoption of a person-centred approach to dementia care. In Britain, the leading publication in the field, the *Journal of Dementia Care*, has run a series of articles devoted to person-centred care and in the January/February 1997 edition, for example, the term is to be found on the contents page in relation to five different articles.

I would freely count myself amongst those who view this trend as positive and I share an enthusiastic optimism about the potential impact of the person-centred tradition on the overall quality of dementia care. At the same time, I must also admit to a growing unease at an emerging tendency for many new, thoughtful and innovative developments in dementia care to lay claim to being person-centred. There is a danger of the phrase becoming synonymous with 'good quality', and of any new approach to dementia care being obliged to identify itself as being person-centred in order to avoid being dismissed as old fashioned, or as partially neglectful of the human aspects of care. I therefore hope that this initial look at the meanings we might intend to convey when using the term 'person-centred' will prove to be timely.

The Meanings of 'Person-Centred'

My awareness of the extent of the diversity of meanings that have become attached to the expression 'person-centred' was greatly increased when I witnessed the reaction of a Person-Centred Therapist who had just read one of the case studies in the *Journal of Dementia Care's* 'Person-Centred Care' series. Her astonishment at the lack of resemblance to the theory and practice that constitute her own work was matched only by her bemusement as to why the term 'person-centred' was being used at all. For her, the term 'person-centred' is the accepted successor to 'client-centred' in referring to the therapeutic approach developed and articulated by Rogers. In practice, it refers to a trained, skilled therapist using their understanding and awareness of their own self in harmony with a conscious use of the 'core conditions' (described below) in order to enable a client-led process of change. She would recognise, of course, that in addition to his work on psychotherapy, Rogers devoted attention to many other areas of life in which human relationships play a central role. These included education, group conflict, group leadership and family life — areas in which he sought, somewhat tentatively, to extend the application of his theories of therapy and of the human personality. She would also, however, point out the strength of the theoretical link between his ideas in these different areas (for example, Rogers, 1959) and how this work was very much an extension of his theory of therapy, being phrased very much in the same language and utilising the same constructs. There is relatively little problem, then, in understanding why we might describe his work in these areas (and that of his successors) as being person-centred.

Problems of understanding do arise, however, as a result of the term 'person-centred', and its various derivatives, coming to be used with a great deal more elasticity, in a host of different settings in which the Rogerian influence is clearly present, albeit in a more diluted, less obvious, form. Thus we have educational methods being described as 'student-centred', social services departments aiming to be 'user-centred', even trade unions resolving to be 'member-centred'. No doubt the authors of many of the articles describing person-centred dementia care are making an equally indirect, even unconscious, acknowledgement of the principles developed by the founder of Client-Centred Therapy. It seems appropriate, therefore, to begin our attempt to unravel some of the plurality of meanings that are being given to the term 'person-centred' with a brief account of the ideas that characterised the work of Carl Rogers.

Carl Rogers: Theory of Personality and of Therapy

The reader of any historical guide to Rogerian psychotherapy may well draw the conclusion that his therapeutic practice flowed naturally and coherently from his theoretical ideas. This appearance is something of a distortion, encouraged by hindsight, as the relationship between theory and practice was, in fact, reversed. It was the many years of clinical experience that shaped Rogers' theoretical outlook, 12 years' experience of working with psychologically disturbed children and a further 20 years working with adults, prior to the publication of the hugely popular *On Becoming a Person* (1961).

Theory of Personality

The approach developed by Rogers constituted a radical break from both the behaviourist and the psychoanalytic traditions which had, until then, formed the most influential attempts to understand human behaviour and the development of human personality. He had experienced a growing awareness that the principles which grew out of, and then informed, his own therapeutic endeavour were quite distinct from the Freudian beliefs expressed by many of his contemporaries. As these principles became more fully articulated, it became clear that the view Rogers was developing was opposed to

Freudian views on the characteristics of human nature, views which Rogers saw as being fundamentally negative and pessimistic. By way of contrast, Rogers argued: 'In my experience I have discovered man to have characteristics which seem inherent in his species, and the terms which have at different times seemed to me descriptive of these characteristics are such terms as positive, forward-moving, constructive, realistic, trustworthy' (Rogers, 1957a, p200).

This 'forward-moving' tendency was not, for Rogers, the sole preserve of the human species. His youthful fascination with agriculture had left him with the seeds of his later belief that all life forms were subject to an observed, directional force — the 'actualising tendency' — towards maturation, improvement, self-maintenance and self-protection. In the 'human organism' this tendency is directed not only towards meeting those needs which are related to our survival as a species — safety, nourishment, shelter and reproduction — but also towards those 'higher' aspirations such as learning, creativity, seeking pleasure and the forming of relationships.

The actualising tendency is a key construct in Rogerian theory. Its status as the sole 'drive' or 'motivational force' present within the human organism leads us naturally to question how Rogers explains the many problems that can occur in the development of a human personality. Whereas Freud posited the existence of destructive drives, or forces, to explain such difficulties, Rogers developed an account based on the processes involved in the formation of an individual's personality and on the 'structures' that these processes produce. One process central to his theory is that of the symbolisation of experience into consciousness, or into awareness. 'Experience' is described as the totality of those sensory and internal processes or events that are present within an organism and which could, potentially, be available to consciousness. As consciousness would be overwhelmed by the volume of experience that is available to it at any one time, the organism must select (from the mass of raw data) and 'symbolise' that part of experience which is allowed into consciousness. Such symbolisation can be accurate or distorted, or it can involve varying degrees of denial, depending on the relationship of the experience to another key construct, the 'self-concept'.

Rogers argued that humans do not possess a self-concept prior to that point in infancy at which they achieve the capacity to conceptualise themselves as distinct, individual entities and to distinguish between their own experiences and a separate 'reality'. Before reaching this point, infants unerringly value experiences that they like and they attach negative values to experiences that they dislike or which threaten them. They have an 'organismic valuing process' which will allow them, for example, to hit out when they feel angry and also to accurately symbolise the experience into consciousness: 'I hit out because I was angry and that is OK.' Soon, however, the infant reaches the stage in which they begin to form a self, or self-concept, an: ' ... organized, consistent conceptual gestalt composed of perceptions of the characteristics of the "I" or "me" and the perceptions of the relationship of the "I" or "me" to others and to various aspects of life, together with the values attached to these perceptions' (Rogers, 1959, p200).

For Rogers, it is a characteristic of the formation of the self that it is accompanied by the development of a need for 'positive regard'. If this need is satisfied, it will allow the self-concept to be grounded in a perception that the individual is valued by others. This, in turn, will be internalised as 'positive self-regard'. If the infant perceives that it predominantly and consistently receives positive regard from significant others (usually, though not exclusively, the parents) that is not contingent on its own behaviour, then it is said to experience such regard as being 'unconditional'.

More commonly, however, parents will manipulate, or be perceived by the infant as manipulating, the dispensation and withholding of positive regard in order to bring about desired behaviour in the infant. They will show disapproval when the infant hits out and, depending on the clarity of the message and the interpretative abilities of the infant, this may be perceived as a threat to withhold positive regard. The infant may not be able to distinguish, for example, between the intended message 'I do not like the behaviour of hitting out' and other possible interpretations: 'I do not like you because you hit' or 'I do not like you because you become angry'. Positive regard is thus perceived by the infant as being 'conditional' and this sets up conflict between the infant's organismic valuing process (the satisfaction of hitting out when angry) and the need for positive regard. Such is the need for positive self-regard (based on positive regard from others) that the latter will often win out, resulting in the infant having either to distort or to deny to consciousness the satisfaction it experiences in hitting out when angry. It may be that the satisfaction is denied to awareness altogether, or that its symbolisation into consciousness is distorted so as to take on the value attributed by the source of regard, and so the infant begins to perceive the behaviour of hitting out as unsatisfying. Thus the value — or the 'condition of worth' — which the infant perceives as being attributed to the experience by the parents actually becomes that of the infant. It has become internalised, or introjected, as imposing a condition of the positive regard that the infant needs. This will, if consistently repeated, become a conditional feature of the individual's self-regard in future years.

Through processes such as these, the symbolisation of experience into consciousness becomes less reliable and a degree of 'incongruence' develops between organismic experience and the self-concept. If, as a result of this discrepancy between the organism and the self-concept, significant experiences are not symbolised into the gestalt of the self-structure, psychological tension results. The individual is subjected to an inexplicable anxiety and an alienation from their 'true' feelings. Such incongruence between organism and self is present, to a greater or lesser extent, in all individuals other than the hypothetical 'fully functioning person'. In extreme cases, in which a large number of conditions of worth have been internalised, almost all of the self-concept is based on valuations that have been taken over from other people. Here the person is totally reliant on others for making value judgements, completely lacking in faith in their own judgemental abilities and thus constantly looking to, and anxious about, the views of others as a source of approval. Rogers described people in this state as having an 'external locus of evaluation' and they stand in contrast to those fortunate individuals who are able to combine a positive self-regard with relatively few internalised conditions of worth, inducing faith in their own organismic valuing and an 'internal locus of evaluation'.

The externalisation of the locus of evaluation will have consequences throughout adult life. Positions which involve responsibility for decision making will tend to be avoided and the perception of the qualities of those who do make decisions will be greatly exaggerated. Life partners may be chosen according to their willingness to act as a source of external evaluation, perhaps reinforcing a poor self-concept and setting up a cycle of negative regard. Equally, there will be consequences for relationships with therapists and with carers, with an exaggerated tendency for the individual to develop dependency on others as a result of their lack of confidence in their own capabilities.

Theory of Psychotherapy
An understanding of this basic structure of Rogers' theory of human personality should help us to appreciate some of its implications for his theory of psychotherapy, most commonly expressed in terms of the 'Nineteen Propositions' (Rogers, 1951). The intended outcome of psychotherapy is described in the fifteenth proposition: 'Psychological adjustment exists when the concept of the self is such that all the sensory and visceral experiences of the organism are, or may be, assimilated on a symbolic level into a consistent relationship with the concept of self' (Rogers, 1951, p513). This optimal position is reached when there are no internalised conditions of worth which lead to some experiences being denied to awareness, thus creating an incongruence between self and organism. Where such incongruence exists, however, there is hope that it can be reduced. The seventeenth proposition asserts: 'Under certain conditions, involving primarily complete absence of any threat to the self-structure, experiences which are inconsistent with it may be perceived, and examined, and the structure of self revised to assimilate and include such experience' (ibid., p517).

The 'certain conditions' referred to here are those described in Rogers' article entitled 'Necessary and Sufficient Conditions of Therapeutic Personality Change' (Rogers, 1957b). They have become widely known as the 'core conditions' but before we look at these in more detail we should take note of the first proposition, that: 'Every individual exists in a continually changing world of experience of which he is the center' (Rogers, 1951, p483). This proposition locates Rogers within the phenomenological school of psychology. Unlike both behaviourism, which either minimises or discounts the role of subjective experience as a causal factor in behaviour, and the psychoanalytic school, which interprets such experience as the product of other, less accessible, psychological forces, the phenomenologist sees the subjective perception of reality as being the prime causal agent of behaviour and, as such, the starting point for any theory of behaviour, personality or therapy. As expressed in the seventh proposition: 'The best vantage point for understanding behavior is from the internal frame of reference of the individual himself' (ibid., p494).

The importance accorded to the perceptions and subjective experiences of the individual implies a different kind of relationship between client and therapist from that which we might expect in work based upon either behaviourist or psychoanalytic principles. If perceptions are the very material through which therapeutic change is to occur, and if it is self-evident that nobody could possibly be more familiar with such material than the individual who experiences it, then it follows that the 'expert' in any therapeutic relationship must be the client themselves. For Rogers, this conclusion is reinforced by the view that each individual's innate actualising tendency will, in the right conditions, translate the knowledge derived from this expert status into the best possible course of action. As two recent exponents of the client-centred approach have summarised: 'The central truth for Rogers was that the client knows best. It is the client who knows what is hurting and in the final analysis it is the client who knows how to move forward' (Mearns & Thorne, 1988, p1).

The therapist abandons the role of expert in Client-Centred Therapy and assumes a role which is commonly described as 'facilitative'. It is probably more accurate to say that Rogers saw the therapist as being an expert in the role of companion, in being able to use their own self to create the conditions necessary to enable the client to initiate change. Thus, rather than attempting to direct the client, or to interpret their experiences, the therapist's energies are devoted to creating the core conditions which Rogers consistently maintained were 'necessary and sufficient' for therapeutic change to occur.

9

The core conditions, drawn from Rogers' own clinical experience, were that for therapeutic change to occur, the therapist must be congruent, accepting and empathic.

Congruent

The therapist must be perceived by the client as being 'genuine' and this will only happen if the therapist has a high degree of congruence between their own organismic experience and self-concept. There can be no disguising their own organismic experiences behind a professional facade, by attempting to adopt the 'role' of therapist. Any incongruence is likely to be picked up by the client (as an inconsistency between the therapist's verbal and non-verbal behaviour) and will undermine the therapeutic relationship.

Accepting

The therapist must satisfy the self-concept's need for unconditional positive regard if experiences which are inconsistent with the self are to be allowed into awareness. Acceptance needs to be shown of the things the client says, does and experiences, of their qualities and of the stage that their self-concept has reached in the process of its development. The therapist must resist any temptation to put their own words or interpretation on to the experiences of the client, even if this interpretation is felt to be more accurate than any the client is currently capable of. The whole point of the therapeutic endeavour is for the client to be enabled to work to this position themselves. Thus the therapist does not contradict the client who is, for example, still at the stage of blaming themselves for suffering sexual abuse in childhood, notwithstanding the incongruence that this might induce in the therapist.

Empathic

The therapist will enter as fully into the client's frame of reference as possible, whilst maintaining a clear sense of their own identity. This enables them to accompany and support the client in their exploration and reconstruction of their inner world and to assist in the client's discovery of their own inner resources.

'Person-Centredness'

Client-Centred Therapy involves a deliberate attempt to create a new balance of power, control and responsibility between therapist and client, a 'democratisation' of the relationship which became a feature that Rogers applied to his work on other areas of human relationships. It would, therefore, need to be included in any list of qualities which we might use to judge claims that a particular approach is person-centred. His thoughts on education, for example, involved a similar transformation of the relationship between teacher and student. Students were best served, in Rogers' view, by being assisted to develop their own potential and by being allowed to assume a large degree of control of, and responsibility for, the content of their studies. The teacher should abandon the role of expert, dispensing the knowledge and skills they have decided the student needs, and adopt that of facilitator, encouraging and supporting the student while eschewing control of the direction of the learning process. Rogers practised much of what he preached in his occupancy of a professorship at Chicago University from 1945 and whilst his methods may have caused much consternation among his colleagues who were steeped in traditional, directive, teaching methods, it is true to say that half a century later student-centred teaching methods dominate much of the world of educational thought.

What other features might form part of our list of person-centred qualities? Below are some of the essential features of Rogerian thought which could be included.

1 A respect for the subjective experiences, perceptions and inner world of the individual, based on the belief that to understand an individual requires us to be familiar, through empathy, with that inner world and to view things as they do: in Rogerian terms, to enter their frame of reference.

2 A non-judgemental acceptance of the unique qualities of each individual, including the stage that the process of their personality development has reached.

3 An emphasis on seeing the person 'as a whole'.

4 A positive view of human nature and its tendency to fulfil its potential.

5   An elevation of the importance attached to feelings and emotions — particularly the need for positive regard — as opposed to cognitive features.

6   An accent on the importance of interpersonal relationships and on the influence that such relationships have on an individual's ability to develop towards their potential.

7   An acknowledgement of the need for authenticity in such relationships.

8   A non-directive approach: an emphasis on the role of the professional as an enabler or facilitator; acceptance that power, control and responsibility remain with the individual.

Implications of Person-centred Principles for Dementia Care

There is some irony in the fact that the greatest resistance to the spreading influence of Rogerian thought has been mounted in the very field — mental health — in which it originally appeared. Rogers was well aware that his views on the role of the therapist, and of the qualities required to fulfil that role, would be viewed as a threat to, and generate opposition amongst, those whose status and self-concept are based on an image of the therapist as a detached expert. His emphasis on the personal qualities of the therapist, as opposed to the amount of knowledge acquired in extensive training, carried a direct threat to the hegemony of the medical profession within psychiatry. This threat is still effectively resisted to this day, as psychiatrists continue to dominate services for the 'mentally ill' and Client-Centred Therapy is marginalised, largely to the (often lucrative) world of the private sector, catering primarily for those that the medical profession dismisses, somewhat insultingly, as the 'worried well'.

The aforementioned spread of person-centred principles has, however, created a pressing need to clarify their implications for dementia care, a clarification which must include an acknowledgement that these ideas, whose origins lay in the treatment firstly of children and their families and then of cognitively intact adults, will require some modification if they are to become meaningful in the context of older people in the process of losing many of their mental powers. As a tentative first step, it may be worth looking at the eight features of 'person-centredness' described above and considering their applicability to dementia care.

Entering Another's Frame of Reference
Attaching central importance to the inner, phenomenological world of the individual has profound implications for the way in which we relate to people with dementia. Whereas Reality Orientation, with its behaviourist foundations, focuses on the functioning of the person with dementia, the person-centred approach is eager to address their experience. Apparently bizarre or confused speech and behaviour, previously regarded as the meaningless outcome of a disease process, challenges the person-centred carer to gain an understanding of the meaning behind such speech and behaviour. It requires them to gain insight into the perceptual world of the person with dementia and of the sense that they are making of reality.

Holding such a position does not require us to form an opinion about the reality of the disease process, or about the nature of its effect on the perceptions. Rather it requires us to acknowledge that an awareness of this causal role will necessarily be of little practical use to our attempting to overcome the barriers to the formation of relationships based on mutuality and contact between the therapist and client.

Non-Judgemental Acceptance of the Unique Aspects of Each Individual Person
Losing some of the abilities that have been present since childhood enhances the need for unconditionally positive regard. People with dementia need more than an acceptance that they are blameless for the consequences of failing powers if they are to maintain a reasonable degree of self-regard. They also require that those around them continue to see them as much more than a set of symptoms of a clinical condition, manifested in a body from which the former occupant has departed. The prevalent view of dementia as the disease which destroys the person and leaves the body behind is incompatible with the need for others to continue to recognise individual uniqueness — a recognition not only of the singular constellation of qualities that make up each person, but also

13

of the highly individualised way in which they react to their predicament. We must maintain the person, as opposed to their illness, at the forefront of our awareness and respect the sense that they make of their situation.

Seeing the Person 'as a Whole'
A fuller appreciation of the qualities of each person will lead us to see beyond their illness. It will enable us to be aware of their strengths, as well as their disabilities, and to concentrate our efforts on maintaining and celebrating those strengths in addition to attempting to mitigate the effects of the disabilities.

Person-centred care of older people with dementia will prize each individual's history, their unique life story. This is not to diminish their present by accentuating their past but rather to acknowledge that each person's present identity is a function of their past, and that reinterpretation and re-evaluation of one's past life is an essential part of revising the self-concept.

A Positive View of Human Nature
There are real difficulties involved in applying the principles contained in Rogers' accounts of the actualising tendency to the traditional view of dementia. His emphasis on the organism's movement towards greater independence and self-responsibility seems at odds with the increased dependence which habitually accompanies dementia. Similarly, there are problems in identifying the potential effect that cognitive impairment can have on the individual's movement through the 'Seven Stages of Process' of therapeutic personality change (Rogers, 1961, p125).

We might want to offer a less restrictive view of the actualising tendency (might not the acceptance of dependency needs be seen as a form of growth?) and point to the way that decline in cognitive function can be accompanied by the preservation, or even enhancement, of other human characteristics. There are numerous anecdotal examples of individuals who have become more emotionally expressive in dementia, as if the dissolution of their (cognitively based) self-concept has allowed them greater access to their own organismic experience.

Whilst dementia may set limits on what may be achieved, a person may continue to seek knowledge, to achieve objectives and to move forward, even if it is within a fragmentation of experience and with a purpose that is not apparent to others.

The Importance of Feelings and Emotions
Many of those who work and live with people with dementia have seen in the person-centred approach the prospect of a liberation from preoccupation with the cognitive aspect of the deterioration which accompanies the disease. The extent of the research into the neuropathology of the disease, while undoubtedly fully justified, serves to highlight the poverty of research and thought on the quality of the emotional lives of people with dementia. The growth in concern for how people are actually feeling, which accompanies the person-centred approach, can have a valuable humanising effect on services that were previously delivered in a somewhat cold and impersonal manner. Dementia care that claims to be person-centred has to have at its heart a concern with emotional well-being. It will also acknowledge, validate and respond to expressions of grief, fear, alienation, anger, bitterness and other painful emotions which are natural accompaniments of the experience of dementia.

The Importance of Interpersonal Relationships
Following on from this concern with emotional well-being there must be an acknowledgement that it is only through genuine psychological contact with other people that such well-being can be promoted. As people lose their ability to maintain contact through language there is a proportionate increase in the need to maintain contact and communication through non-verbal means. Person-centred dementia care places a strong emphasis on the maintenance of good quality, warm, human contact through whatever methods of communication are appropriate. It also wants to understand the ways in which people with dementia form and maintain relationships of trust and affection, with caregivers and with each other, despite the decline in their powers of memory, powers which might have seemed to be a fundamental prerequisite to the formation of trust.

The Value of Authenticity in Relationships

There are grounds for arguing that the person whose experience is sharpened as a result of being 'uncluttered' by memory, and by the cognitive understanding of that memory, may be in a better position to discern any incongruence that others may bring to relationships. Similarly, a decline in the ability to comprehend verbal communication means that the person with dementia becomes increasingly reliant on their ability to react to non-verbal cues. It is therefore all the more incumbent upon caregivers to ensure that their non-verbal communication is unambiguous, and that it is received as such.

A Non-Directive Approach

Person-centred dementia care will aim to maximise the autonomy of individuals and to enhance their feeling of being in control of their actions and their daily lives as far as is possible. Whilst there will be obvious constraints, there will also be an appreciation of the need to maintain a sense of agency and a willingness to adapt environments in pursuit of this aim. The provision of environments which facilitate a non-directive approach is perhaps the biggest design challenge facing those who organise the care of people with dementia.

In interpersonal terms the person-centred approach leads us to the position whereby we are obliged in our conversations with people suffering from dementia to encourage them to set the agenda. We do this by being receptive to the expression of the current concerns, regardless of their factual status, and by being willing to accompany the sufferer from dementia in their exploration of those concerns.

Ways of Being in Person-Centred Dementia Care

In the same way that attempting to reduce the art of Client-Centred Therapy to a series of techniques is to entirely miss the point of Rogers' message, there is a danger that extracting some of the key features of the wider person-centred approach will fail to do justice to the role of the caregiver in dementia. Elusive concepts such as 'a way of being' with those who require our help may be grasped on an experiential level whilst their defiance of definition leads to their being overlooked in theory. Rogers held that the theoretical model and associated techniques of the therapist were of less importance than their attitude and how this attitude was conveyed to the client. His summary of the attitudinal qualities was framed as a series of questions in an attempt to explore the question, 'How can I create a helping relationship?'

1 Can I be in some way which will be perceived by the other person as trustworthy, as dependable or consistent in some deep sense?

2 Can I be expressive enough as a person that what I am will be communicated unambiguously?

3 Can I let myself experience positive attitudes toward this other person — attitudes of warmth, caring, liking, interest, respect?

4 Can I be strong enough as a person to be separate from the other?

5 Am I secure enough within myself to permit him his separateness?

6 Can I let myself enter fully into the world of his feelings and personal meanings and see these as he does?

7 Can I be acceptant of each facet of this other person which he presents to me?

8 Can I act with sufficient sensitivity in the relationship that my behaviour will not be perceived as a threat?

9 Can I free him from the threat of external evaluation?

10 Can I meet this other individual as a person who is in process of becoming, or will I be bound by his past and by my past? (Adapted from Rogers, 1958)

It is encouraging to note that these questions require no modification or reinterpretation if 'he' is a person who is suffering from dementia. This is indicative of their relevance to all human relationships, to their 'humanness', and we might conclude that, whichever approach we espouse, if we are able to answer these questions positively then we are in a position to give truly person-centred dementia care.

CHAPTER 2

Validation Therapy

A S CARL ROGERS WAS DEVELOPING the ideas that have come to have such a marked influence on the way many in the western world viewed human personality and relationships, the daughter of a neighbouring Midwest state, Naomi Feil, was growing up in the Montefiore Home for the Aged in Cleveland, Ohio. Her father, a psychologist, worked as the administrator of the home which also employed her mother as a social worker, so when Feil left to study psychology and social work at Columbia University, New York City in 1950, she was following in the footsteps of both parents. On completing her studies in 1956, she remained in New York as Director of Group Work Services in both a hospital and a community centre, working with a client group that she has since described as the 'oriented, healthy elderly' (Feil, 1992a, p9). She also took up acting in 'Off-Broadway' theatre.

In 1963, two years after the publication of Rogers' *On Becoming a Person* (Rogers, 1961), Feil returned to the Montefiore Home and began work as a group therapist. In her first published article (Feil, 1967) she describes her earliest attempts at groupwork with residents who were selected on the basis that they were neither engaging in the organised groups and workshops provided by the home nor making any social contact with residents, staff or others from outside the institution. These 'outcasts', as Feil describes them, were divided into two groups according to their 'ego strength' and their consequential 'ego contact with reality' — according, as we might say now, to the degree of their disorientation. In both groups the therapeutic endeavour was termed 'remotivation' and the Montefiore Home's emphases on rehabilitation and on mitigating the effects of institutionalisation were well to the fore.

This first article is noteworthy in three respects: for its arguments against attempting to orientate more disorientated group members; for the messages it gives us about the growing Rogerian influence on Feil's practice; and for containing the first clues about her views on the processes at work in creating disorientation (a holistic 'theory of disorientation', incorporating psychodynamic elements, that has been the source of some puzzlement regarding Feil's understanding of the dementing process and, consequently, regarding her ideas as to who may benefit from the use of Validation).

Abandoning Attempts to Orientate Group Members

Although Feil described her early groupwork with disorientated older people as 'remotivation', it is clear from her 1967 article that this approach had close links with the principles behind Reality Orientation (RO), which was gaining widespread acceptance in the USA following the pioneering work of Dr James Folsom in Alabama. Holden and Woods (1982) have described how remotivation groups with members diagnosed as having senile dementia employed methods similar to RO. Both were strongly influenced by behaviour modification and were 'highly structured and [made] use of objective topics of conversation and visual aids ... with positive feedback for accurate statements being made explicit' (Holden & Woods, 1988, p48). They also shared some of the same goals: 'in terms of improved interest, awareness etc' (ibid.).

Feil's experience of using groupwork with those who had a low level of 'ego contact with reality' left her unimpressed at the efficacy of remotivation with this population. After three years, she came to the conclusion that 'Bringing in objective material ... did not work with this group. They could not move from themselves objectively to the outside world. Each one was trapped in a world of fantasy' (Feil, 1967, p194). She later confirmed that 'My initial goals [in 1963] were to help severely disoriented old-old to face reality and relate to each other in a group. In 1966, I concluded that helping them to face reality is unrealistic' (Feil, 1992a, p9).

Feil shared with Rogers a tendency to confront theoretical issues primarily as an attempt to make sense of experience gained in clinical practice. Her search for an alternative approach did not result from a shift in her theoretical viewpoint, it was, rather, an outcome of her frustration with the failure of existing therapies to benefit those who had passed beyond a certain level of disorientation: 'I came to realise that the goal of reality orientation was in itself unrealistic. After six years of failure to bring about awareness of time, place, age, recognition of staff or family relationships' (Feil, 1972a, p3).

Feil continued to acknowledge the potential therapeutic value of RO when it is used with people whose disorientation is relatively mild. These individuals, who she would later describe as 'malorientated', often have both the desire and the ability to be orientated to reality. When an individual has passed beyond this stage, however, the continued use of RO becomes futile at best. Indeed Feil came to feel that the very goals of RO may be undesirable: 'In 1969 I found that not only was awareness of reality intolerable for this group of aged whose reality held steady deterioration in functioning, loss of affectional ties, and whose future held death; but sudden insight into reality brought about pain, withdrawal, and increased dependency' (ibid.). She illustrates the point with the example of a group member whose 'paranoid diatribes against the administrator' of the home had, on one level, sustained him for five years until he 'suddenly realised that his accusations were not realistic'. As a result of this insight:

He stopped talking, and gave up his cane for a wheelchair. His physical deterioration, coupled with the loss of the fantasy which had given him strength, changed his self-image. He needed his fantasy to maintain himself. His hatred of the administrator was his life-preserver. He is now impassive in the group, his head drooping in his wheelchair, his eyes sad and empty of fight.
(Feil, 1972a, p3)

Whilst we may question whether these 'paranoid diatribes' were truly a form of disorientation (in that it would be highly unusual for sudden insight into disorientation resulting from cognitive impairment to occur after five years) we can observe that, by 1972, Feil had become convinced that those who have lost ego contact with reality will resist attempts to orientate them. This resistance is mounted, in her eyes, with good reason and, should it be overcome, the result may well be detrimental. She had thus moved beyond the increasingly common criticism that RO becomes merely ineffective once the level of cognitive impairment removes the possibility of its success.

The Influence of Rogers on Feil

There are parallels between Feil's movement from an awareness of the limitations of the dominant therapeutic approaches to the creation of an alternative theoretical framework and Rogers' own journey from frustration with the contemporary orthodoxies (psychoanalysis and behaviourism) to the formation of a new school of humanistic thought. Given that Feil was setting out in the period in which Rogers' ideas first gained mass circulation, it is not surprising that his ideas would have some influence on her attempt to create a new approach to working with people with dementia.

Feil's earliest articles, written between 1967 and 1972, reveal a growing acceptance of the need for the therapist to address the subjective experience, the 'inner reality', of disorientated group members. In Rogerian terms, she was arguing that empathy, entering the group member's 'frame of reference', must be the starting point for therapy: 'Only relevant exploration of subjective feelings ... could stimulate group members' (Feil, 1967, p194); 'Through entering the inner world and bringing the inner reality outward — residents can experience each other and feel like somebody' (Feil, 1972b, p3); 'In verbalising the 'fantasy' or inner reality, individuals gained a feeling of gratification, of being understood, and a sense of self in the knowledge that their world was meaningful and acceptable' (Feil, 1972a, p6).

This phenomenological influence was not provided by Rogers alone. Feil also reports the influence of the existentialist 'anti-psychiatrist' R.D. Laing, whose *The Divided Self* (Laing, 1960) convinced many people involved in mental health of the inadequacies of the dominant 'medical model' of psychiatry. The 1960s saw a flowering of approaches challenging the claim to 'objectivity' made by a psychiatric profession which attempted to explain mental health problems as if they were analogous to physical diseases. Where the psychiatrist aspired to objectivity, the anti-psychiatrist criticised them for 'objectification': for describing minds as if they were subject to the same type of processes as organs of the body. The revolt against psychiatry emphasised our subjective, experiential existence and stressed the fundamental differences between the nature of 'mind' and the nature of 'matter'. It drew support from the existentialist philosophers whose popularity had burgeoned in Europe during the years following the Second World War and whose ideas formed one of the many different intellectual focal points of the 'counter-culture' which swept through advanced capitalist countries during the latter part of the decade.

In developing her own approach, Feil combined this respect for the subjectivity of her group members with an increased concern for their emotional well-being — a shift which required her to re-evaluate the objectives and priorities of groupwork. The result was a move away from cognitive or behavioural targets towards affective goals, stressing the centrality of the quality of the relationship between therapist and group member:

Our goal is to reawaken a feeling of self-worth through self-awareness and accomplishments; to reduce emotional pain, to promote interaction between one human being and another, and to teach the staff to enter into the inner world of resident, so that staff can relate with empathy, treating individuality instead of lumping these residents as 'dead wood'.
(Feil, 1972b, p1–2)

This is the earliest published example of Feil using 'empathy' to describe a central aspect of the relationship between therapist and group member. Another of Rogers' core conditions, regard, can be discerned in the claim that the relationship will be strengthened by: 'the worker's demonstration that he is aware of the assets of the individual' (Feil, 1967, p195).

By the early 1970s, Feil had made a sufficiently radical departure from existing methods of groupwork with people with dementia to justify her using the title 'A New Approach to Group Therapy with Senile Psychotic Aged' in her address to the 25th Annual Meeting of the Gerontological Society in 1972 (Feil, 1972a). In the following years Feil teamed up with her husband to produce a series of short films promoting the new approach, now also being developed as an interactive skill for use with individuals. Her confidence in the pertinence of Rogerian principles to her client group was such that in the 1978 film, 'Looking for Yesterday', she asserts that only an approach (described then as 'Tuning-In Therapy') based on a willingness to enter another's frame of reference can hope to benefit the 'severely disoriented aged'.

The worker's ability to empathise is seen as a fundamental requirement if they are to 'tune into the inner reality of the disoriented aged' (Feil, 1978, p4). The need for congruence is highlighted: 'Empathy does not permit a patronising tone of voice' (ibid., p2) and later expanded upon: '[Validation] workers never run behind by patronising and pretending. They know the disoriented old are wise and recognise the pretender ... Disoriented old-old have intuitive wisdom. With failing eyesight they 'see' who patronises them. With dim hearing they 'hear' the pretender' (Feil, 1982, p4). And the third core condition is included: 'Through acceptance of feelings, each person gains a sense of identity and belonging in this world' (Feil, 1978, p4).

These person-centred features of Feil's work were carried forward into the development of Validation Therapy (initially known as Validation/Fantasy Therapy) which appeared in 1982 with the publication of her first book, *V/F Validation: The Feil Method*. Despite the apparent continuity, however, it is at least arguable that Tuning-In Therapy has a more credible claim to being a person-centred approach than Validation Therapy, which superseded it. For the new elements in Feil's theory that appeared between 1978 and 1981 — the four stage model of disorientation, the modified version of Erikson's life-stage theory, and the theory of symbols — owe little to the traditions of humanistic psychology. Indeed the appearance of such elements were examples of Feil's willingness to incorporate concepts derived from dissimilar — often seemingly incompatible — sources including, in the latter two cases, concepts which have their roots firmly in the psychoanalytic tradition.

Psychodynamic Influences on Feil

Feil's Views on Disorientation and on Dementia

Feil's disillusionment with existing therapeutic approaches combined with a cynicism induced by the contemporary diagnostic confusion surrounding disorientated older people — she cites one individual who received five different 'labels' between 1963 and 1971 (Feil, 1982, p9) — to persuade her to abandon her attempts at directing disorientated older people and to begin, in her own words, to listen to them instead. During the same period she began to gather anecdotal evidence, largely through discussion with relatives, that much of the speech and behaviour of disorientated older people which had previously been dismissed as meaningless actually made some sense if the listener had sufficient knowledge of the resident's earlier life. Feil began to reject the idea that the kind of 'global' disorientation which involves people re-experiencing situations and relationships from the distant past is a pathological process: that is, the result of neurological damage which renders individuals unable to remain orientated. She began to understand it as the outcome of a type of psychodynamic process, involving a return to significant psychological points from the past in order to resolve unfinished emotional conflict.

Thus, whilst the Rogerian approach to psychotherapy certainly helped to shape the changes Feil initiated in her practice as a group therapist, it was largely to the psychoanalytic tradition that she turned when she attempted to formulate a new theoretical account of the processes which lead to the development of disorientation in later life. Thus began a marriage, considered uneasy by some, that has lasted to the present day.

The resistance that group members showed to Feil's early attempts to orientate them resulted, in her eyes, from the prevailing tendency to dismiss confused and disorientated speech as meaningless, and therefore not worthy of a response. Failure to attend to the apparently confused articulations of group members' current concerns created barriers which Feil was determined to break down. In responding to disorientated people on their own terms, without threatening the validity of their perception of reality, she was beginning to work within the broad tradition of humanistic psychology. But she did feel it was not enough to simply accept, to 'be with', people in their disorientation. She also saw a need to understand, to interpret, their confused speech and behaviour. Her earliest writings show her optimism regarding the feasibility of this task: 'I used the approach that all behavior, no matter how bizarre, had a rational explanation' (Feil, 1967, p194).

By the time she produced the first edition of *V/F Validation: The Feil Method* (1982), this 'approach' had become a fundamental tenet, listed as a 'basic belief' in the book's opening paragraph: 'There is reason behind all behavior' (Feil, 1982, p1). For Feil that 'reason' must exist, because behaviour, no matter how bizarre or disorientated, is never simply the scrambled output of a damaged central nervous system. Her belief is that the 'disoriented' speech and behaviour we witness in 'the disoriented old-old' can best be understood as the outpourings of a psyche that is no longer bound by social or internalised constraints.

Thus, from her earliest writings, Feil is not working from an orthodox, reductionist 'medical model' view of dementia, a view which posits that the disorientation which accompanies a dementing illness — in all its behavioural and cognitive aspects — can be wholly explained in terms of (and is therefore caused by) a neuropathology. Although this rejection was not fully articulated until later writings, she proceeds even at this early stage with an assumption that 'circulatory and organic brain syndrome' is but one amongst many factors which can contribute, in varying degrees, to generate disorientation or, to use Feil's early phrase, to people having 'lost ego contact with reality [and] regressed to an almost infantile level of behavior' (Feil, 1967, p194).

Other contributory factors would include elements of the physical: 'severe arteriosclerosis accompanied by … strokes, tumours, gastric disturbances, and … urinary disturbances' (ibid.); personal history: 'All except one were housewives with narrow prescribed role expectations and little education' (ibid.); and the social psychology of the institution: 'an intense dependence upon the motherly nursing staff' (ibid., p195). (Indeed, it is the latter which is identified as the greatest single obstacle to group therapy achieving its goal of increasing the independence of group members.)

Feil summarises this interplay of factors which leads to severe disorientation thus:

> gradual organic deterioration and subsequent loss of physical and psychic controls; the process of disengagement in ageing and consequent loss of social roles, status, spouse, friends; separation from children; the dependent qualities inherent in institutional living, all combined to create a loss of ego contact with reality and regression to early modes of self-gratification.
> (Feil, 1972a, p2)

More recently, Feil and her daughter, Vicki de Klerk-Rubin, have emphasised that impaired vision and other sensory deficits can be significant contributory factors in bringing about disorientation, and they have also paid more attention to the role played by Alzheimer's Disease and other primary dementias. In the case of Alzheimer's Disease, they point to the fact that the hallmark neurofibrillary tangles and neuritic plaques have been found in the brains of individuals who were fully orientated when alive and they use this as evidence to support their belief that disorientation is not a necessary result of the disease. Some old-old people, Feil asserts, can suffer the same neuropathology found in Alzheimer's without showing signs of disorientation. The crucial difference between these 'oriented old-old' and their disoriented counterparts is, she states, the course that their personality development has taken throughout their earlier lives, and particularly the degree of success with which they coped with Erik Erikson's developmental life tasks (to be discussed in the next section). Feil sees the disoriented old-old as being those who have failed to progress satisfactorily through Erikson's stages and who have, as a result, been left more susceptible to becoming disorientated on two counts: firstly, their earlier difficulties will have left them with tendencies (especially towards denial and repression) which render them unable to face the losses of old-old age and, secondly, they have a need to return to those earlier stages in order to complete the unfinished life tasks, and to resolve the past crises, before they die. For these are the people who 'have denied severe crises throughout their lives' (Feil, 1992a, p27).

Thus, although Feil and her supporters will agree that there are organic diseases of the brain which can cause problems with memory and orientation, they will also argue that in the population which can be helped by Validation, the disoriented old-old, disorientation is not a necessary result of the disease. In this population, disorientation is held to be best explained in psychodynamic terms, hence Feil's early use of 'Fantasy' as an alternative phrase.

Who is Validation Therapy for?
A widespread misunderstanding of Feil's idiosyncratic views on the nature and causation of disorientation has encouraged the growth of some confusion over the target population for Validation. Indeed, some authors have expressed doubts as to whether she intends Validation to be used with people with dementia at all. Stokes and Goudie, for example, state that Validation is: ' ... not appropriate for people suffering from Alzheimer's Disease or multi-infarct dementia, with the possible exception of when the dementia is in the earliest and therefore mildest stages' (Stokes & Goudie, 1990, p182), whilst Tom Kitwood complained that: 'the proponents of Validation Therapy have tended to be vague about the applicability of their ideas to those who have a primary degenerative dementia' (Kitwood, 1992, p23).

The confusion clears, at least to some extent, with the realisation that Feil is not defining the group which might benefit from Validation with reference to dementia (or any other biological/disease phenomena) as we might anticipate. She defines the 'disoriented old-old' in terms of their level of disorientation which, as we have seen, she understands primarily in (Eriksonian) developmental terms. In later writings, Feil compounded the confusion by identifying the disoriented old-old as those with 'late-onset dementia' (Feil, 1992b) and 'Alzheimer's-type dementia' (Feil, 1993) but these apparent concessions to orthodoxy should not obscure the point that, for Feil, a significant determinant of the occurrence of disorientation is the individual's history of personality development, as much as any plaques, tangles and/or infarcts in their brain. In conversation on this point, Feil does acknowledge that, in some old-old people, cognitive impairment may be the predominant factor, as it is with younger people with the disease. For the majority, however, disorientation (while still perhaps the product of a multiplicity of factors) is primarily the result either of an Eriksonian regression or of the need to escape (by denial) from an unbearable present reality.

Thus we can summarise Feil's position as a psychodynamic theory of disorientation. She sees disorientation in the old-old as a coping mechanism for dealing with an unbearable reality and also as a regression to previous, unfinished, developmental stages. This is not to deny the possibility that neurological damage is one of the factors which provokes its use, albeit as a defence mechanism for the psyche: 'Denial of reality has become a coping mechanism for these aged. Holding on to the past helps them survive. Their future and their present is living day after day, feeling useless in a nursing home' (Feil, 1978, p2).

The ideas deployed in support of Feil's position do have currency in other circles. They tend to focus on perceived gaps in the empirical evidence, especially the weakness of correlation between, in the case of Alzheimer's Disease, the neuropathology observed on post-mortem and the degree of clinically observed disorientation during life. There is insufficient evidence, it is argued, to justify the belief that disorientation is a 'symptom' of the disease. Steve Scrutton, for example, has spoken of the 'social creation of confusion' and he echoes Feil's thoughts when he states:

> there are many features of social life which might be instrumental in creating, developing and reinforcing confused mental states. Their impact is to make the lives of many older people unbearable, so unbearable in fact that they become unwilling to retain contact with the present realities.
> (Scrutton, 1989, p175)

Feil does not deny the existence of organic brain disorders, nor does she claim to be providing any kind of 'cure' for them when she claims that the successful use of Validation can, on occasion, result in improved orientation. If disorientation is seen as a reaction to dementia, as opposed to a symptom of it, then her claims that Validation achieves improvements in orientation, mood and behaviour should be viewed as claims that it is helping people to adjust to damaged brain cells and other losses, not as claims that it is reversing the symptoms of dementia. Part of this adjustment means that 'Some disoriented old-old no longer need fantasy when they feel strong and worthwhile in present time' (Feil, 1982, p3). In this sense, then, she is making the same type of claim as that being made by the other authors whose work is discussed in this book. Where Validation differs from other approaches, however, is in the extremely limited degree of influence that its adherents are prepared to grant to neuropathology as a causal factor in producing disorientation. A publisher's note at the beginning of Feil's 1993 book, *The Validation Breakthrough*, declares:

> The subtitle of this book, *Simple Techniques for Communicating with People with 'Alzheimer's Type Dementia'*, may be confusing to some readers. As used here, the term Alzheimer's-type dementia is intended to include people in their late 70s or older who have lost some recent memory; who have some sensory impairment; and who have been diagnosed as having senile dementia of the Alzheimer's type, dementia or Alzheimer's disease. Some people diagnosed as having Alzheimer's disease may not actually be suffering from the disease. A definitive diagnosis of Alzheimer's disease is possible only on autopsy, when the brain of the deceased person is inspected for plaques and tangles. Dementia or disorientation is often caused by a multitude of factors other than Alzheimer's disease, including some loss of memory, eyesight, hearing, work, family, and friends.

Whilst this note may generate more questions than it answers (for example, what is causing the memory loss, if not Alzheimer's?), it is clear from its final sentence that, according to this view, disorientation may result from a combination of biological and non-biological factors or even from a combination of non-biological factors alone. It is also worth noting that Feil and de Klerk-Rubin use the term 'dementia' to describe a collection of symptoms as opposed to its more common usage as an umbrella term for a number of disorders, the most common of which is Alzheimer's Disease.

The ground we have now covered should leave us in a somewhat better position to understand the list of characteristics with which Feil summarises the 'disoriented old-old' — that group who may benefit from Validation:

Disoriented old-old are very old people who:
• have inflexible behaviour patterns
• hold on to outworn roles
• have to grapple with unfinished feelings
• withdraw from present day reality to survive
• have significant cognitive deterioration and can no longer function intellectually to achieve insight.
(Feil, 1992a, p26)

---

and:

Validation helps people who:
1. are old-old, aged 80–100 plus.
2. have led relatively happy, productive lives.
3. have denied severe crises throughout their lives.
4. hold on to familiar roles.
5. show permanent damage to their brain, eyes, ears.
6. have diminished ability to move, control feelings, remember recent events.
7. meet their human needs for love, identity, and expression of feelings by using body movements and images learned early in life.
(Feil, 1992a, p27)

Feil's Addendum to Erikson's Psychosocial Developmental Stage Theory
In 1992 I attended a one day workshop on Validation Therapy presented by Naomi Feil at London's Queen Elizabeth II Conference Centre. She began by asking delegates to raise their hands if they had small children which I, having a daughter who was three years old at the time, dutifully did. As I was sitting in one of the front rows I was selected by Feil and asked to describe some of my daughter's behaviour, how she would play with dolls and speak to them as if they were her own children, how she

would act out scenes in which she imagined that she was much older than she actually was, perhaps set in some faraway place. Was I worried by this behaviour? Did the fact that my daughter was acting and talking as if she were in an 'unreal' situation lead me to seek a psychiatric assessment, perhaps requiring some cognitive testing? Of course not. The audience's laughter indicated that the point had been made. The reason I need not worry about my daughter's behaviour was that I knew it to be appropriate to the developmental stage she had reached. So it is, Feil declared, for the disorientated old-old. If disorientated speech and behaviour in a 50-year-old should properly cause us some alarm, in those over 80 it should be seen as perfectly natural, because they are in the 'Resolution versus Vegetation' stage of life.

In the early 1980s, at the time that the term 'Validation' was first used to describe her approach, Feil attempted to graft the ideas of the psychoanalytic theorist Erik Erikson on to her account of the process of disorientation in the 'old-old'. Erikson's model of personality development consists of a series of developmental stages, which he described as the 'eight ages of man' (Erikson, 1950), each of which is characterised by a particular developmental 'task' or 'crisis'. In earliest infancy, for example, the task is to develop a sense of trust. To carry out this task successfully an infant will require the gratification of oral needs and a reasonably consistent and satisfactory response from the primary caretaker (usually the mother) to its expressions of need. If these conditions are met, the infant will develop the ability to trust and to hope. If they are not met, the tendency to mistrust will be carried forward into the next developmental stage.

Throughout Erikson's model the prospects of successful transition at each stage are influenced largely by interpersonal elements (key relationships), the outcome of previous stages and (with growing significance) the availability of useful role models from the stage that the individual is moving towards. The model is summarised in Table 1.

Feil accepted Erikson's model in its entirety but felt it necessary to make one addition so as to extend its applicability to the disoriented old-old:

Table 1 *Erikson's 'Eight Ages of Man'*

Developmental Stage	Psychosocial crisis
First Year	basic trust v. basic mistrust
Toddler	autonomy v. shame and doubt
Early Childhood	initiative v. guilt
Middle Childhood	industry v. inferiority
Adolescence	identity v. role confusion
Adulthood	intimacy v. isolation
Middle Age	generativity v. stagnation
The Ageing Years	ego integrity v. despair

Source: Adapted from Erikson (1950, pp222–243).

Erikson defined the final goal of lifespan development as being that of achieving 'ego integrity or despair'. This seems too global to be useful for work specifically with the disoriented elderly, and so for the purposes of using the Validation approach, a ninth stage has been added; that of 'resolution versus vegetation'.
(Feil, 1992b, p204)

The influence of psychodynamic theory, which had earlier encouraged Feil to find meaning in apparently confused speech and behaviour, now, through this adaptation of Erikson's model, persuaded her that disorientation also had a purpose. For Feil, the concept of disorientation had been transformed from being a tragic consequence of an irreversible and progressive disease process to being a necessary and productive endeavour to resolve life's past crises, and so to begin preparations for death. It is easy to see the potential appeal of this transformation for caregivers, both professional and family, who are faced with the demoralising prospect of the inevitable deterioration of the person they are caring for. In addition to inspiring hope, Feil's reframing of the process provides a positive role for caregivers, that of assisting the disorientated old-old in moving towards resolution. The caregiver, who had previously seen their role as giving comfort during a process of terminal decline, now had a positive therapeutic role to play: that of enabling the accomplishment of the final life task.

The introduction of the concept of the final life stage allowed supporters of Validation to distinguish between the disorientated old-old (whose disorientation is understood in developmental terms) and the younger person with Alzheimer's Disease whose disorientation is a result of the neuropathology and who cannot be helped by Validation. De Klerk-Rubin draws this distinction between the 67 year old 'true Alzheimer's patient' and the disorientated old-old person:

> Both would be described as SDAT (senile dementia of the Alzheimer's type) if they failed the standardized tests. The behaviour is not so different, but the reasons behind the behaviour are quite different. Our 67-year-old man is a good example of what Naomi Feil ... calls the young disoriented or true Alzheimer's patient. The 'demented' behaviour doesn't fit with the life stage. (de Klerk-Rubin, 1994, p14)

Feil believed that the need to add a further stage to Erikson's model resulted from his failure to take account of the growing population of old-old (from around 75 to 80 years and upwards) people, many of whom are disorientated in a way that Feil believes is not pathological. Erikson, primarily concerned with child development, included only one stage in old age ('Integrity versus Despair'). Feil argues that this may be sufficient to describe those who have achieved integrity, and have no need to return to resolve issues from the past, but that, in order to include those who still have unfinished business from earlier life, her final stage is needed: 'Resolution versus Vegetation'.

Feil's Theory of Symbols

I referred earlier to one of the basic beliefs behind Validation: that 'There is reason behind all behaviour' (Feil, 1982, p1). Thus far we have concentrated our attention on Feil's efforts to discern the reason, or meaning, behind confused and disorientated speech. Speech is, of course, just one aspect of behaviour that can appear to be confused, bizarre or meaningless. Those who have spent any length of time with people with dementia are aware that many other behaviours can appear purposeless and without meaning, especially if the person does not have the verbal capacity to explain their actions.

Using ideas derived from both Freud and Jung, Naomi Feil claimed that an understanding of the meaning behind such actions is made possible by a kind of 'universal language' of symbols used by disorientated people whose verbal communication becomes impaired. This language consists of the use of certain types of objects which come to symbolise either objects or people from the person's past or more generalised 'internal objects', or archetypes, which Feil described as 'universal longings'. Careful observation of the disorientated old-old person will reveal a pattern to the use of certain objects as symbols, either as universal longings:

A napkin becomes the earth. Neatly, carefully, meticulously, an old-old woman ... folds, caresses, pats, croons, kissing each fold. She is putting herself in place. She is putting herself in order on this earth. She *belongs*. She is happy. Her world is in order. The napkin is her ticket to express her longing to be *loved*.
(Feil, 1982, p42)

---

or as personal memories: 'A purse symbolizes a filing cabinet for a former file-clerk. She files, filling her purse with Kleenex. The Kleenex become vital documents she folded as a legal secretary' (ibid.).

Feil held that 'confused' behaviour, previously written off as little more than a symptom of the neuropathology of Alzheimer's Disease, can in fact be understood and interpreted as a series of symbolic actions which reflect the preoccupations of the unconstrained psyche. A knowledge of the symbols, which are 'universal, regardless of race, religion, culture or sex.' (Feil, 1992a, p49) will assist the caregiver in deciphering the meaning. Reproduced below are Feil's list of universal symbols, formed 'After 35 years of working with maloriented and disoriented people around the world' (ibid., p47).

Universal Symbols and What They Can Mean

Jewelry, clothing	Worth, identity
Shoe	Container, womb, male or female sex symbol
Purse	Female sex symbol, vagina, identity
Cane or fist	Penis, potency, power
Soft furniture	Safety, mother, home
Hard furniture	Father, God
Napkin, tissue, flat object	Earth, belonging, vagina, identity
Food	Love, mother
Drink from a glass	Male power, potency
Any receptacle	Womb
Picking the nose	Sexual pleasure
Playing with feces	Early childhood pleasures
(Ibid., p48)	

Although few would deny that the inner world of disorientated older people may sometimes involve present-day objects being used as symbols in the way that Feil suggests, there is little support for the belief that there is a universal language of symbols and Feil herself now views the idea of such a language as mistaken. Her current view is that the use of objects as symbols actually becomes more idiosyncratic as the degree of disorientation and disability increases.

For all that she was prepared to adopt psychodynamic concepts to assist her understanding of the processes in dementia, the actual approach of the Validation Therapist continued to be based largely on Rogerian principles. The use of symbols, the emphasis on regression and the understanding of the life-stage were all seen as useful tools in assisting the Validation worker in making some sense of the inner world of the disoriented old-old. That understanding however, served only to facilitate the development of empathy, and it is clear that the 'balance of power' in the therapeutic relationship continues to bear the hallmarks of a person-centred approach. The initiative remains firmly with the client: 'Empathy does not mean analyzing. The V/F worker validates the right of feelings to exist. Empathy means acknowledging feelings that the person freely expresses. Validation does NOT mean exploring feelings that the person chooses not to express' (Feil, 1982, p3).

We will look at how successful Feil and the supporters of Validation have been in their attempt to amalgamate the diverse, even opposing, outlooks of the psychodynamic and person-centred traditions when we have completed our exploration of the other key theoretical foundations of her approach.

The Four Stages of Resolution

When Feil, de Klerk-Rubin and other proponents of Validation employ the term 'disorientation' they intend a meaning that is quite different from its orthodox meaning. Whilst there may be common understanding on the observable phenomena known as disorientation, there is a contrasting interpretation of its origins and nature. Most people involved in dementia care understand disorientation as one of the symptoms of the disease. As such, they would expect that, broadly speaking, disorientation will, along with other symptoms, become more severe as the disease progresses. They might acknowledge that the rate of increase in the severity of the various symptoms will vary from one individual to another, as will the relative severity of the different symptoms, but nonetheless there is a general consensus that most of this variation can be explained in terms of the differing neurological terrain in which the same neuropathology — or group of neuropathologies — is operating. Anyone who shares this conceptualisation of dementia will tend, therefore, to assume that when Feil gives a description of 'the stages of disorientation', she is describing something similar in character to, or perhaps parallel to, a traditional model of 'the stages of dementia' (for example, Hughes *et al*, 1982). This assumption would itself rest on the conviction that Feil accepts that the movement through the stages of disorientation will, like movement through the stages of dementia, be both progressive and irreversible.

It is this erroneous assumption that has led many to misinterpret Feil's claims that the use of Validation may arrest, even reverse to some degree, movement through the stages of disorientation as implying a claim that it can arrest the progress of a dementing illness (this is, perhaps, one of the reasons why they were renamed 'The Four Stages of Resolution' with the publication of *The Validation Breakthrough* in 1993).

Feil developed her four-stage model of disorientation at the same time as she was adapting Erikson's life-stage theory and both have become defining features of Validation Therapy. In her 1992 'definition' of Validation, Feil states firstly that it is 'a way of categorising the behaviours that are exhibited by the disoriented elderly into four discrete and progressive stages' (Feil, 1992b, p200). The nature of the link between the 'Resolution versus Vegetation' life-stage and the Four Stages of Disorientation is a little unclear. Renaming them the 'Four Phases of Resolution' — and describing each as a 'substage' of Resolution versus Vegetation — seems to imply that progression through the stages is a positive process, in that it involves the individual moving towards the achievement of resolution. But movement through the stages is, in fact, held by Feil to be a negative development, ending not in resolution but rather in its counterpoint, 'vegetation'. The aim of Validation is to prevent movement from one stage into another, using the techniques which, as we shall see later, are appropriate to each stage. A summary of Feil's 'Four Stages of Disorientation' is provided in Table 2.

Stage One: 'Malorientation'
Feil's 1993 book *The Validation Breakthrough* includes an account of four characters, each of which is described as being 'maloriented'. All four are referred to as being 'blamers' and their shared characteristic is that they are well orientated but that they 'repeat one thing that is often not true in terms of present-day reality' (Feil, 1993, p64). This 'one thing' is typically a false accusation about some current figure in the life of the maloriented person. Upon investigation, it becomes clear that the maloriented person is wrestling with some unresolved crisis from an earlier life stage. Unresolved feelings towards a significant individual from that crisis are still present and are now being transferred to an unwitting victim from the present or to some fictitious, metaphorical character who encapsulates the essential emotional flavour evoked by the crisis. The cognitive state of the maloriented person is unclear, for while Feil asserts that all four individuals were 'diagnosed as being in the early stages of Alzheimer's disease, with paranoid delusions and hallucinations' (ibid., p68), a list of the physical [sic] characteristics of maloriented people states that

Table 2 *Feil's Four Stages of Disorientation*

	Stage One Malorientation	Stage Two Time confusion	Stage Three Repetitive motion	Stage Four Vegetation
Basic helping clues	Use who, what, where and when questions Use minimal touch Maintain social distance	Use 'feeling' words (I see ..., I feel ...) Use touch and eye contact	Use touch and eye contact Pace to person's movements	Mirror movements Use sensory stimulation
Orientation	Keeps time Holds on to present reality Realizes and is threatened by own disorientation	Does not keep track of clock time Forgets facts, names and places Difficulty with nouns increases	Shuts out most stimulation from the outside world Has own sense of time	Will not recognise family, visitors, old friends or staff No time sense
Body patterns: muscles	Tense, tight muscles Usually continent Quick, direct, movement	Sits upright but relaxed Aware of incontinence Slow, smooth movements	Slumped forward Unaware of incontinence Restless pacing	Flaccid No effort to control continence Little movement

	Purposeful gait		Slow, steady	Frequent finger movements
Vocal tone	Harsh, accusatory and often whining	Low, rarely harsh; Sings readily		
Eyes	Clear and bright; Focused, good eye contact	Clear, unfocused; Downcast, eye contact triggers recognition	Eyes usually closed	Eyes shut, face lacks expression
Emotions	Denies feelings	Transfers memories and feelings from past to present situations	Demonstrates feelings openly	Difficult to assess
Personal care	Can do basic care	Misplaces personal items often	Cannot care for themselves	Cannot care for themselves
Communication	Communicates clearly	Begins to use unique words	Mainly non-verbal	None readily apparent
Memory and intellect	Can read and write	Can read but no longer write legibly	Is not motivated to read or write	Difficult to assess
Humour	Some humour retained	Unique humour	Laughs easily, often unprompted	None readily apparent

Source: Adapted from Morton & Bleathman (1988, pp25–7; Feil, 1992a, pp108–9).

'Their recent memory is largely intact, although occasional lapses occur' (ibid., p64) and 'Their cognitive abilities, including the ability to tell time, remain intact' (ibid.).

It is much easier to understand how such 'maloriented' people might come to be described as having paranoid delusions, as the examples quoted do involve persistent false beliefs which are unresponsive to reason or evidence and which are of a persecutory nature. Many of the people, or 'composites of real people' (Feil, 1993, p51), would, I suspect, be seen as having the type of encapsulated delusions that have, in Britain at least, often been associated with a diagnosis of 'paraphrenia'.

Whilst maloriented individuals are held not to be suitable for Validation Groupwork, owing to their low tolerance for expressed emotion and discussion of feelings, Feil does state that sufficient individual Validation can prevent an advance towards the next stage.

Stage Two: 'Time Confusion'
We are likely to find the person Feil describes as 'time confused' rather more recognisable as someone who will attract a diagnosis of Alzheimer's Disease or one of the other dementias. They correspond in many ways to those commonly described as having a 'moderate' degree of dementia, in that they are usually disorientated in time, place and person, retain some long-term memory whilst having but have a profoundly damaged short-term memory. They are still able to communicate verbally but have some word-finding difficulties and a tendency to create neologisms, and they require some assistance with personal care and other activities of daily living.

Validation was developed with this group in mind. It is the time-confused who 'retreat from reality to escape from boredom and a bleak present-day reality and relive familiar scenes from the past, which they often struggle to resolve' (Feil, 1993, p84). It is suggested that this group, along with those from Stage Three, will benefit from both individual and group Validation.

Stage Three: 'Repetitive Motion'
The most noticeable indication that an individual has moved to Stage Three, 'repetitive motion', is the onset of marked dysphasia, as the

ability to use and understand language is lost and sounds start to be made for pleasure and/or stimulation. All the skills required for daily living are either absent or under threat, as are the internalised inhibitions that control the expression of emotion or the satisfaction of needs: 'Feelings that have been stopped up for a lifetime, now overflow. The plug is gone' (Feil, 1992a, p54).

Stage Four: 'Vegetation'
This final stage corresponds with 'severe dementia'. Individuals have become unresponsive, inactive and immobile. Feil suggests that Validation may be attempted on an individual basis with this group, but acknowledges that this is more in hope than in any realistic expectation of achieving a therapeutic effect.

Movement between the Four Stages
Feil states that, whilst some may move between the first three stages from moment to moment, most people can be located as being in one particular stage most of the time. She is clear in her belief that sufficient Validation will prevent deterioration to the next stage, as progression to the next stage is characterised by a further withdrawal inward, either to escape reality or to deal with an unresolved life-task. As Validation makes reality more tolerable and assists in the resolution of old conflicts, the tendency to withdraw inwards should reduce and a willingness to face reality increase.

Other Theoretical Aspects of Validation

A look at the reference lists in Feil's publications reveals a host of influences other than those mentioned here. The main influences on the development of Validation have undoubtedly been Carl Rogers, along with Abraham Maslow, from the humanistic tradition and Erik Erikson, along with Freud and Jung, from the psychoanalytic tradition. It should also be added that the tremendous impact that Robert Butler's work on Life Review had in terms of redefining reminiscence as a normative aspect of ageing (Butler, 1963) was also influential, as were Piaget's accounts of the pre-linguistic use of movement and self-stimulation in children (especially in the understanding of people in stage three, 'repetitive motion'). The theory of the 'preferred sense', which is discussed in the section on Validation techniques, appears to have its origins in the theory behind Neuro-Linguistic Programming.

Reflections and Comments on Validation Theory

At her 1992 Validation workshop in London, Feil revealed that 'the practice was developed first, the theory came later'. A review of her publications since 1967 shows that, whilst her singular view of disorientation and dementia was evident from the beginning, it was only at the end of the 1970s, as the theory and practice of Validation was developed, that Erikson's life-stage theory was incorporated and the Four Stages of Disorientation were introduced.

As Feil grew increasingly frustrated with the perceived limitations of the efficacy of remotivation and RO, she clearly felt that approaches which fail to address the subjectivity of the individual will create barriers between the therapist and the disorientated person. RO has received a great deal of 'bad press' in recent years, much of which has resulted from practitioners using it in an insensitive and mechanistic manner. Rather like a poor teacher who maintains a psychological detachment while churning out endless information, some practitioners have seen RO as a therapy requiring a minimum of intellectual and emotional effort. Indeed, this disengagement, which so often blights the progress of interpersonal 'techniques', became a characteristic of much of the culture that grew up around RO during its period as the dominant therapeutic approach to working with dementia. This was much to the chagrin of its most significant proponents, who campaigned for its use as a highly individualised technique and who mourned the demise of its lost companion, Attitude Therapy, which could have mitigated against the development of such a culture (for example, Holden & Woods, 1982, p52).

Her account of the criteria used in the selection of members for her earliest groups indicates that Feil has never made distinctions on the grounds of cognitive functioning (Feil, 1967, 1972a) and it is worth noting that both RO and remotivation were, at this time, not prescribed solely for those diagnosed as having 'Organic Brain Syndrome' (Holden & Woods, 1982, p50; Feil, 1993, pp131–132). Indeed, there appears to have been a great deal of classificatory confusion around the diagnosis of dementia, which led to Feil's complaint:

> To add to the confusion, labels change about every ten years. From 1963–1971, Mr. Smith's label changed five times for the same behavior and the same laboratory findings. He was labeled: Arteriosclerotic, Senile Demented, Ambulatory Schizophrenic, Senile Psychotic, Organically brain damaged, chronic. In 1970 hundreds of disoriented old-old were labeled 'Senile Demented'. In 1981, the same people with the same undetermined number of degenerated clumps of nerve fibres viewed through a CT scan, were labeled Alzheimer's Diseased.
> (Feil, 1982, p9)

The evolution of Feil's theory has to be understood in this context. She rejected RO and related behavioural approaches for this population because she saw them as dismissive of the things that disorientated people were actually saying: they failed to listen and they 'wrote people off'. She saw the diagnostic process around what we now call dementia as being discredited. It was constantly changing and Feil could see that the effects of labelling — awareness of which had grown throughout the 1960s with the influence of Goffman's work — was another way of writing off disorientated people. Determined to counter these damaging trends, Feil made what she saw as being a series of necessary counter-assertions: that disoriented people must be listened to (with empathy, the influence of Rogers) because their speech and behaviour has meaning (influenced by Laing, Freud and Jung). Later she was to reinforce this position by claiming that even the most disorientated speech and behaviour not only has meaning, it also has purpose (on a developmental level, the influence of Erikson).

The growth in the international popularity of Validation was symptomatic of the widespread dissatisfaction at RO's inability to fill the therapeutic void in dementia care. According to Feil's own figures, that growth has seen the use of Validation spreading from 523 homes in the USA and Canada (Feil, 1982, p12) to over 7,000 institutions worldwide (Feil, 1993, pxi) in little over a decade. But, whilst many would share her reservations about RO, with even its erstwhile supporters agreeing that 'the techniques of RO can be used to demean, devalue and patronise' (Woods, 1992, p126), and others express support for her resistance to the negative effects of diagnostic labelling (for example, Kitwood, 1990a), yet still there is a significant reluctance to accept the theoretical foundations of Validation — especially its account of the nature of disorientation and dementia.

Issues Raised by Feil's Theory of Dementia and Disorientation
Feil argues that the 1981 decision of the American Psychiatric Association's *Diagnostic and Statistical Manual* task force on nomenclature and statistics to abandon the distinction between senile and pre-senile dementia was unhelpful, in that it has drawn attention away from the fundamental differences in the way that Alzheimer's Disease affects younger and older sufferers. She accepts that in younger sufferers (approximately 70–75 and under) it is reasonable to assert that the observed psychological and behavioural changes are caused by the neuritic plaques and neurofibrillary tangles that are the neurological hallmarks of the disease. In older people (75–80 and over — the disorientated old-old), however, the situation is complicated, in Feil's view, by at least four factors which should serve to undermine our confidence in the primacy of the role played by neuropathology.

1 Neuritic plaques and neurofibrillary tangles have been found in the brains of people who died in old-old age without showing any signs of disorientation or other symptoms of Alzheimer's Disease when alive. There is a looseness in the correlation between the post-mortem examination of the brain and clinical features observed during the lives of the older age group.

2 The old-old commonly suffer from a multiplicity of physical factors which can contribute to disorientation. Feil lists increased sensory deficits, impaired circulation in the brain and accumulated neuronal loss as being particularly significant, whereas in younger sufferers Alzheimer's usually appears in the context of generally good health.

3 The increase in losses suffered by the old-old renders them more likely to utilise disorientation as denial, acting as a defence against an unbearable reality.

4 The process of personality development is such that, when old-old people are disorientated, it is, in an Eriksonian sense, age-appropriate behaviour as the individual may be involved in the task of resolution which is crucial to the successful completion of the (final) life stage.

These complicating factors lead Feil to assert that 'The anatomical structures that change the brain and are seen at autopsies, are not the sole orchestrators of behavior at very old age. The condition of the brain is rarely the answer to the behavior of the living old person' (Feil, 1992a, p31). Feil may well be justified in highlighting the potentially complex nature of the inter-relationships between factors that can bring about disorientation. It should be pointed out, however, that, if the research evidence which would allow us to infer a direct causal connection between neuropathology and disorientation is inconclusive, how much more so is the evidence connecting disorientation with factors 2, 3 and 4 above. To be consistent, Feil surely has to be even more tentative about the causal role of these factors than she is about the plaques and tangles. Does an individual's history of personality development influence their prospects for becoming disorientated? We can suggest, at most, that this may be a possibility, but when Feil accounts for those old-old people who have remained oriented despite features of an Alzheimer's type neuropathology, she is very clear that it is variables pertaining to personality and behaviour that have been the determining factors in preventing disorientation:

Neurofibrillary tangles and senile plaques are found in the brains of all people with Alzheimer's disease. They are also found in many people who do not exhibit any signs of dementia ... Many people over 80 survive damage to these brain cells and remain oriented ... these people retain the ability to communicate verbally, are aware of present time and place, and are able to make appropriate judgements. These people have:

- Faced the challenges and disappointments of their lives
- Tackled the problems of daily living with a sense of hope
- Forgiven themselves and others for their mistakes and failures
- Compromised when they could not fulfill goals
- Continued to respect themselves despite failures, mistakes, and dreams that were not fulfilled
- Survived physical and social losses
- Accepted their physical deterioration, loss of loved ones, and inevitable death
- Maintained a zest for living
- Avoided dwelling on the past, but enjoy reminiscing
- Established new relationships
- Prepared for death by making peace with their loved ones

(Feil, 1993, pp21–22)

The proponents of Validation cannot reasonably ask us to reject the evidence in support of the claim that neuropathology causes disorientation and then ask us to accept that factors such as those listed here by Feil can prevent it — an acceptance that would be based on substantially less evidence. This is not to deny the possibility of a multiplicity of causal factors combining to induce disorientation in very old people, it is rather to admit that currently we can have very little justified confidence in our ability to identify the degree of influence that each of these factors might have in any one case.

It is also difficult to support the compatibility of Feil's apparent willingness to accept that the behaviour of younger people (those under 75) who are diagnosed as having Alzheimer's Disease is explicable purely in terms of their neuropathology: 'Brain damage alone in a younger person often relates to behavior' (Feil, 1982, p9). De Klerk-Rubin (1994) carries this distinction between the 'true Alzheimer's patient' and the 'Disoriented old-old person' to its logical conclusion. If the plaques and tangles do not necessarily lead to disorientation in old-old age, and if the presence of disorientation is contingent upon other, perhaps reversible, factors then it follows that, whereas a characteristic of the 'young disoriented or true Alzheimer's patient' is that he or she 'deteriorates no matter what caring method is used' (de Klerk-Rubin, 1994, p14), the disoriented old-old person 'can improve, will not necessarily continue to disorient' (ibid., p15).

Whilst we may wish to applaud Feil and de Klerk-Rubin's insistence that we should not allow diagnostic labelling to lead us to 'write off' disoriented old-old people, they clearly fail to account adequately for this difference in prognosis between the 67-year-old 'true Alzheimer's patient' and the 80-plus-year-old 'disoriented old-old person'. Why should the same neuropathology be an (irresistible) causal agent in the younger person and not in the older person? De Klerk-Rubin's suggestion is that the answer lies in the 'huge physical, psychological and social changes that take place in those twenty years. It a 67 year old man becomes lost in the neighbourhood he has lived in for forty years it is for a different reason than if an 87-year old loses her way in her own house' (ibid., p14).

In other words, it is the accumulation of non-neuropathological characteristics that occur in this twenty-year period. Yet, surely, this is a matter of degree. A 67-year-old still has sixty-seven years of accumulated characteristics. Assuming that the rate of accumulating characteristics is constant, the 67-year-old's prospects of resisting the consequences of the neurological changes should be 77 per cent of those of the 87-year-old. Given their generally superior health, there appears to be no logical justification for the 67-year-old being inevitably condemned to suffer the fate meted out by Alzheimer's Disease, whereas the 87-year-old is held to have the potential to resist it.

A far more coherent position for the supporters of Validation to adopt would be to accept that the influences on the course taken by Alzheimer's Disease are multifactorial in individuals at all ages and to acknowledge that there is a real neuropathology which is producing real cognitive deficits. To make such a move necessitates neither writing people off nor denying the potential for psychodynamic or person-centred interventions, any more than it would when working with people with any other mental or physical disability. Again, in conversation Naomi Feil is happy to accept that there are some old-old people who are disorientated as a result of changes that have occurred in their brains, as well as those who are disorientated as an escape or as an Eriksonian regression. For her, the primacy of practice greatly reduces the significance of such theoretical issues, leading her simply to advise: 'If Validation helps – use it, *regardless of the label!*' (Feil, 1982, p9).

It should also be pointed out that supporters of Validation are irritated by a tendency, particularly strong in Britain, to evaluate it as if it were a specific treatment to be used with people with a particular illness. Their belief that the disorientated old-old are not ill means that their claims really are more along the lines of 'This is a helpful way to be with people who are at this stage of life', as opposed to 'This set of interventions will improve these particular aspects of people with this particular condition'. Whether one accepts that the people they describe as the disoriented old-old are 'people at a particular stage of life' as opposed to 'people with a particular condition' is contingent upon whether one accepts Feil's adaptation of Erikson's model of personality development.

Issues Raised by Feil's Adaptation of Erikson's Developmental Theory
We have seen that Feil's search for the meaning and purpose behind the behaviour of people with dementia was fuelled by the widespread tendency for these people to be written off by others. It led her to reframe the orthodox view of disorientation, now seen as the key to a new life-task, and this, in turn, committed her to rejecting the idea of disorientation as a symptom of a disease. Our ability to follow the process behind the development of Feil's understanding of dementia does not, however, diminish our awareness of the fact that we are being asked to abandon the notion of disorientation as a symptom purely as an act of faith. Only if we accept the notion of the 'Resolution versus Vegetation' life-stage are we obliged to view disorientation in the same way as Feil, and there are some powerful arguments against such acceptance. For the least we could demand of any credible extension to Erikson's model is that it is consistent with the earlier stages, as they were elaborated by Erikson himself. These stages share the characteristics of being universal and sequential: each stage has to be gone through and they must be gone through in the same order. In the case of Feil's addendum (the Resolution versus Vegetation stage), however, it is clear that many people do not become disorientated in old-old age — it is almost a 'second chance' for those who failed to progress through a particular stage first time around.

Those who have managed all earlier stages successfully are fortunate in not having to become disoriented to achieve resolution, but in this Feil's addendum is quite unprecedented in Erikson's earlier stages.

This belief, that disorientated speech and behaviour in old-old age is likely to represent an attempt to resolve a crisis from an earlier psychosocial stage, has led to a curiously narrow band of individual dementia sufferers being described in the literature supporting Validation. Feil and her supporters frequently present vignettes in which confused speech and behaviour are 'decoded' to reveal an individual who is re-experiencing significant scenes and individuals from the past. The behaviour and speech of the people who inhabit these vignettes often remind me of people with dementia that I have known. After reading several such 'case studies', however, I became aware that I was always being reminded of the same few people and that there are many people with whom I have worked who would not fit neatly into one of these vignettes at all. These are people who fit the criteria of being 'disoriented old-old' in that they are over 80, they have significant memory damage, marked communication difficulties, seriously impaired judgement and daily living skills, and are disorientated in time, place and person. What they do not show, however, is a tendency to behave as if they were actually living in the past. They do not know what year it is, or how old they are, but they are not behaving as if they believe they are much younger than they actually are or as if they believed it was many years ago. This characteristic, which I estimate is shared by a large proportion of people with dementia, does not appear in the Validation literature because it does not fit the theory of disorientation. The disorientation is profound and the people affected clearly spend the majority of the time feeling bemused and unsure of their surroundings, yet they have not 'retreated to an earlier reality' nor do they show any sign of having a well-developed alternative interpretation of current reality. There arc, therefore, no indications to suggest that their disorientation may be psychodynamic in origin.

It could be argued that people with a late-onset dementia that is marked by a disorientation showing none of the psychodynamic qualities described in the Validation literature are not truly the disoriented old-old, in that they have not 'denied severe crises throughout their lives'.

They are, the argument may run, quite happy to behave as if they are in present time as they do not have to retreat from reality and they have no unfinished life tasks that they must return to. The problem with this line of defence is that it undermines the key distinction between the 67-year-old 'true Alzheimer's patient' and the 87-year-old 'disoriented old-old' — the twenty-year age gap — which is the justification for denying that the disorientation of the latter is not due to the condition of the brain. We have seen how de Klerk-Rubin is clear that it is the 'huge physical, psychological and social changes that take place in those 20 years' (de Klerk-Rubin, 1994, p14) which justify the assertion that the 67-year-old's disorientation is caused by illness, whereas the 87-year-old's is part of the life stage. This line of argument does not permit the possibility of an 87-year-old whose disorientation is caused by illness.

There are many involved in dementia care who share the impulses behind Feil's attempt to reconceptualise disorientated speech and behaviour in dementia, to transform it from a symptom of a progressive and terminal disease into a positive and necessary attempt to complete life's unfinished business. Despite the empathy we may feel towards Feil's motivation, we have to acknowledge that it is a failed attempt. It does not fit with the logic of Erikson's model to add on a stage through which only a few will need to pass, and it does not take account of the many old-old people with dementia who do not retreat from reality. I do not wish to deny that there are disorientated people who spend at least some of their time re-experiencing significant situations and individuals from their past. With such individuals it may well be appropriate to utilise some of the techniques Feil recommends to assist them in coming to terms with past conflicts. What I cannot accept, however, is that the significant majority of confused speech and behaviour is likely to have this psychodynamic origin, or that we should always look first for this kind of explanation. It was such a belief that led Feil to develop the most contentious of her ideas — the theory of symbols — which has since been abandoned.

Issues Raised by the Four Stages of Disorientation
It was mentioned earlier that the four-stage/phase model of disorientation should not be confused with those stage-specific

medical models of dementia which have emerged in recent years. One major difference is the medical model's assumption that each stage will be passed through (providing the patient lives long enough) and that the only real question is how rapid that process will be. Feil is clear, however, that Validation can prevent people moving from one of her four stages to the next and that it may, in some circumstances, even reverse the process. Thus the editor's postscript to Feil's 1992 chapter is mistaken on two counts when it states:

> It is important to emphasize that, when the four stages of dementia were developed to form the Validation approach in the late 1960s purely on behavioural observations, there were no comprehensive stage-specific medical models of dementia to help clinical research and practice. It is reassuring to see that practical clinical behavioural observations are converging with, and being confirmed by neurobiological advances in understanding dementia.
> (Feil, 1992b, p216)

In fact, the four stages were not developed until around 1980 and it makes little sense to talk of convergence between models that are attempting to encapsulate quite different things. Feil is not attempting to produce a model of dementia. A significant note follows that postscript, referring to a section of the chapter which has been 'inserted by the editor. The author prefers the term disorientation instead of dementia, as used in the title and in several places in the article' (ibid.). Feil prefers the term 'disorientation' because she is not referring to a disease process, nor is she attempting to model the stages of a disease process. Nonetheless, she is trying to categorise the behaviour of the disoriented old-old and the success she has enjoyed in this attempt has been greatly limited by the small sample of people who appear to have been taken into account during the construction of the model. The Four Stages may have been the outcome of 'practical clinical behavioural observations', but whenever I have discussed them with practitioners and caregivers the overwhelming majority find it impossible to fit the disorientated people that they know into any one stage. They commonly say that most people show qualities that are in two, perhaps three, different stages and point out, rightly in my estimation, that to attempt to categorise the behaviour of disorientated people in this prescriptive way is to deny the individuality with which people are affected by dementia. Clearly the success of a four-stage model is compromised if experienced workers in the field cannot place the majority of the people they have worked with into one category rather than another.

On a structural level, there are problems resulting from the inclusion of criteria which Feil acknowledges as being direct results of the disease process alongside others that are held to be independent from it. I refer specifically to the inclusion of memory. I described earlier how Feil writes of memory being damaged by a disease process, just as eyesight, or hearing, might be. If this is the case, memory cannot legitimately be included as being a quality that varies with each stage, as deterioration in memory will be determined by the disease process, unlike the other factors that are represented in the model. In general, Feil speaks of memory being damaged irreversibly, and independently of orientation, yet in the model they are linked. Thus if orientation improves, or ceases to deteriorate, then, according to the model, so does memory — and this is in contradiction to the way that Feil speaks of memory elsewhere.

Perhaps this is to be asking for a degree of precision that the stages were never intended to have. We should recall Feil's telling us that it was the practice that came first, and that the stages were developed largely to help people identify which techniques were likely to be most useful with different individuals. As such they were always something of a 'rough and ready' guide and they should be judged for their utility in this regard rather than as an attempt at an academically credible classificatory system.

Validation in Practice

Had Naomi Feil's approach to working with people with dementia grown out of a previously developed theoretical standpoint, our reluctance to share her views might have led us to dismiss the prospect of finding anything of value in her practice. Fortunately, most of the practice of Validation emerged well before the theory and, although there are aspects of the latter that many find unsatisfactory, this should not deter us from appreciating the innovations in practice for which Feil is responsible. Indeed, only the harshest assessment would fail to acknowledge the significance of the contribution she has made to the advancement of dementia care. Feil predated the next serious attempt to apply person-centred principles to dementia care by over twenty years, a time in which she alone had the courage to insist that we listen to even the most severely cognitively impaired people, and that we treat the attempted communication of each person with the respect that it is due. She swam for many years against the tide of what was fashionable and acceptable in the world of dementia care, when the rest of us were being persuaded that the one cardinal sin is to 'reinforce' confused speech and behaviour by giving it attention. Whilst the majority were thinking solely in terms of functioning and behaviour management, she alone was trying to make genuine contact, and for that she deserves our praise.

Given that Feil's practice predates her theory and that the Rogerian influence was strongest in the early, pre-Validation, days — at the time she first sought to establish a practical alternative to RO — we should not be surprised that those psychodynamic influences which have had such an unfortunate effect on the theory of Validation have had relatively little impact on the practice; a practice which was already well developed before the ideas of Erikson, in particular, were incorporated. There is, however, one significant distortion in practice which results from the psychodynamic excesses of the theory. This is the tendency to concentrate the attention of Validation workers on people who do show disorientated speech and behaviour that appears amenable to psychodynamic interpretation. The Validation literature's case examples are dominated by interactions in which disorientated speech and behaviour respond to Validation by revealing their true nature as re-enactments of significant life events.

In general, however, Feil's tendency to merge a host of different, even incompatible, sources and influences may have left her with a theory that is incoherent and unconvincing but it has not prevented her from generating some adventurous and innovative practice.

Individual Validation
The essence of individual Validation is to be found in its refusal to allow factual inaccuracies, apparent digressions or seemingly

irrelevant material to inhibit the possibility of having meaningful communication with someone with dementia. A common response to this point, especially from practitioners and caregivers who have been used to working with RO, is to ask if this implies that we should agree with the person with dementia who is, for example, seeking to go home to their mother. They might suspect that a Validation response runs in a way something like the following.

Example A

Person with dementia:	'It's time I was going, Mother will have the tea ready by now and will be wondering where on earth I am.'
Caregiver:	'Is it that time already? Your mother will be getting anxious!'

This would not, of course, be considered a Validation response. To think of this type of response as being the only alternative to an orientating response is to remain preoccupied with the issue of addressing the factual inaccuracy. By way of an analogy, I am reminded of how, as student psychiatric nurses, we were encouraged to respond to someone (of any age) who appeared to have a fixed, paranoid delusion. The most helpful response, we were told, to a patient who expresses such a delusion is neither to agree (which would collude with, and therefore reinforce, the delusion) nor to disagree (which might lead either to the patient dismissing us as a fool or to our becoming part of the delusion) but rather to focus on the emotional implications, or accompaniment, of what is being said. A typical interaction may run as follows.

Example B

Patient:	'My next-door neighbour is working for the Mafia. He's been ordered to follow me.'
Nurse:	'You must feel really frightened about that.'

With this example in mind, it might be that our original example would involve a response such as in the following.

Example C

Person with dementia:	'It's time I was going, Mother will have the tea ready by now and will be wondering where on earth I am.'
Caregiver:	'You're worried that she might be worrying.'

This principle of not allowing factual inaccuracies to impede effective communication on the matters of current concern to the disorientated person, can liberate the caregiver from that perceived obligation to orientate which many believe, somewhat misguidedly, constitutes the therapeutic essence of RO.

A parody of the compulsion to orientate, used in workshops by Christine Bleathman, illustrates the exasperation this obligation can generate when she asks workshop attendees to imagine they have just suffered a major emotional trauma and have phoned a friend to elicit some much needed support.

Orientating friend:	'Hi, how are you?'
Traumatised person:	'I'm terribly upset, I had a blazing row with my partner last week and she walked out and I haven't seen or heard from her since. I've just been crying non-stop and now I'm going out of my mind with worry because I just don't know where she's gone.'
Orientating friend:	'Oh that's terrible! When did this happen?'
Traumatised person:	(*sobs*) 'Last Tuesday.'
Orientating friend:	'No it couldn't have been last Tuesday because that's when we went out drinking together and you stayed over here. Don't you remember?'

Traumatised person:	(*sobs*) 'I've been so mixed up, it must have been Wednesday.'
Orientating friend:	'No it couldn't have been Wednesday either because I called you first thing Thursday morning to remind you to take those papers to work, and you were fine then. Remember?'
Traumatised person:	(wails) 'Oh it must have been Friday then! Who cares what day it was?! The point is, what am I going to do? I haven't eaten for days, I can't sleep, I can't concentrate on work and I just keep breaking down and crying. What am I going to do?' (Begins sobbing uncontrollably.)
Orientating friend:	'Do you want to know what I think? I don't think it could have been Friday either because wasn't that the day when your mother was coming to visit and you had to pick her up from the station? You were going out for a meal with her Friday night. Surely you wouldn't have fought in front of your mother, would you? ... Hello? ... Hello?'

(Traumatised Person hangs up and searches for the telephone number of a more empathic friend.)

It is striking, even encouraging, to note how many caregivers have been led by their experience to conclude that repeated orientation with people who are profoundly disorientated can generate more distress than it alleviates. Often such carers have quietly abandoned RO before they attend any workshop on Validation or other alternative approach. Such caregivers are apt to report that they find in Validation 'nothing new', as also observed by Vicki de Klerk-Rubin who reports on the frequent expression 'of relief that there is a name for what they have been doing intuitively' (de Klerk-Rubin, 1994).

Caregivers and practitioners do not necessarily require training in Validation to avoid, or shake off, the habit of automatic orientation and to focus their attention on the emotional needs of the person with dementia. There are, however, specific techniques developed by Validation therapists which, as they are unlikely to arise from 'common sense', do require some training. I should also confess, at this point, that the above introduction to the practice of individual Validation is coloured by the value that I attach to the more person-centred aspects of Validation, as well as by my resistance to those aspects which have psychodynamic origins. Readers would find a stark contrast between my non-directive reflections of the emotional content of what is being said and descriptions elsewhere in the Validation literature in which the caregiver is more actively attempting to establish the factual nature of the past scene in which the disorientated person perceives themselves to be. For the sake of balance, I have summarised one such interaction below.

Nurse:	It looks like you enjoyed your lunch.
David:	I'm so hungry, so hungry.
Nurse:	It looks like you had quite a large lunch and that you ate it all; are you still hungry?
David:	Yes, I'm hungry. I don't have anything to eat, my lunch box is empty.
Nurse:	Why is your lunch box empty?
David:	Because I'm too small, not by much, but I'm too small for what they want.
Nurse:	You don't look very small to me. How is it that you're too small?
David:	I have to carry the plates and for that I'm supposed to be six feet tall.
Nurse:	What are the plates for?
David:	The plates are to build the ships. I have to be six feet tall to work here. Times are tough and they're going to try me for two weeks to see if I can carry them. No pay till then. I'm not six feet, the work is heavy, my wife's at home sick and she hasn't got any lunch either. What am I going to do.
Nurse:	You must have felt very helpless and desperate.
David:	Yes, that's exactly how I feel.

(Adapted from van Amelsvoort Jones, 1985, p20)

Clearly, in this instance the nurse felt that she needed to fill out her own understanding of David's perceptual world before she could address the emotions that were likely to accompany his perceptions. An alternative to this approach might have been to concentrate less on (potentially intrusive) attempts to gain this understanding and to have started with an observation about the way that David appeared, on the basis of his non-verbal communication, to be feeling. It is this tension between validating the disorientated person's feelings and validating their perceptual world which has led to a difference in emphasis, the default line of which originates in the paradox of the person-centred and psychodynamic influences. Whereas the caregiver who leans towards the person-centred approach may be content with focusing on the emotional aspects and with allowing themselves to being led with regard to the perceptual content, those who have picked up more of the psychodynamic tendencies will be concerned to identify the 'past life crisis' which they believe the disorientated person is trying to resolve.

Validation techniques
The Validation worker is encouraged to obtain as much detailed information about the disoriented old-old person as possible: 'The more you know about a person, the easier it will be to use the Validation techniques' (Feil, 1992a, p59). This information, on the person's past history and attitudes to their current circumstances, assists the worker in identifying the 'stage of disorientation' which in turn suggests the Validation techniques that are likely to prove most helpful. It may also point towards those issues which remain 'unresolved' from previous life stages, and so the worker is invited to investigate 'Unfinished life tasks … Unfulfilled basic human needs … unfulfilled ambitions … ways of facing crises … How did [they] face old age losses?' (ibid., p58). Information about important relationships, jobs, hobbies and so on can help to make sense of the behaviour of people in the third stage of resolution, repetitive motion, in which communication becomes more ambiguous.

Feil stresses that the attitude of the therapist, the quality of their attention and the relationships that they are able to develop are crucial if the goals of Validation are to be realised. The 'techniques' which she describes should be employed with this in mind: 'The following techniques are ways to begin a relationship. There is no single formula because every person is different. Each worker must tap his ability to empathise with disoriented old-old' (ibid., p65).

In addition to, implicitly, attaching importance to the core conditions of empathy, congruence and acceptance, Feil has turned to the practice of person-centred counselling for some of the techniques of Validation. These include the following reflective practices:

Rephrasing (for use with people in stages one, two and three): paraphrasing the meaning by repeating key words, especially those which seem to have emotional significance;

Matching the emotion (stages two and three): a physical reflection of the facial expression, voice tone and body posture which demonstrate the emotion that the disorientated person is showing;

Linking (stages two and three): drawing connections between behaviour and an unstated need. Feil identifies three basic needs — to be loved, to be useful and to express feelings. A desire to get home to mother may be serving as a metaphor for a need to be loved, whereas a desire to get home to feed the children may indicate a need to be useful. Making such links may be compared to 'advanced empathy' in counselling skills in that they involve the reflection of that which is only implied;

Mirroring (stage three): this involves a physical reflection of the behaviour of the disorientated person.

Other Validation techniques involve the caregiver using their awareness of their own non-verbal communication in order to enhance their use of interpersonal skills in ways that are widely regarded as good practice dementia care. Validation workers need to show good quality eye contact, appropriate voice tone and the use of touch, which Feil encourages with stages two, three and four. One respect in which Feil's use of touch appears unique is in its use with stage three's 'repetitive movers' in whom, she claims, memories of certain relationships can be evoked, according to where the person is touched.

She lists examples of simple massage-like movements which, according to the part of the body they are used on, will stimulate emotions pertaining to mothers, fathers, lovers, offspring, siblings and pets! Validation workers are also encouraged to use reminiscence and music in informal, everyday interactions.

The techniques for people in repetitive motion are largely non-verbal and even include use of an individualised 'Validation Apron', which:

> has various attachments held on with Velcro, that the elderly person can work with throughout the day. Each apron is created with the individual's needs in mind. For instance, a former waitress would have a pocket filled with napkins for her to fold; a former banker would have a folder filled with play money for him to count; a former secretary would have a pad and pen.
> (Ibid., pp74–75)

There are a number of other techniques which are, as far as I am able to ascertain, unique to Validation. Imaging the opposite (with people in stage one) is used when people are preoccupied with, and agitated by, some (false) injustice or injury. Asking them to elaborate on the times when an alleged injustice does not occur, for example, is designed to assist them in reframing the extent of the perceived problem. Using polarity (stage one) provokes the person into thinking about the worst possible case and thereby hopes to assist in the expression of feelings. Finally, there are three hints at facilitating communication. The first is to use who, what, when, where and how questions (for people in stages one, two and three). It is felt that these closed questions are less threatening than using 'Why' questions which demand more reasoning ability than may be available. The second is to use vague pronouns (stages two and three). When it is not clear who, or what, the disorientated person is referring to, the Validation worker can help maintain the interaction by using vague pronouns. So they might respond to 'I need my X here, I wish X was here' with 'You're missing him, aren't you?' (and watch for signals that might indicate whether 'X' is a 'her', a 'he' or an 'it'). Similarly, when someone uses a vague pronoun themselves, they should not be pressed for identification as this may interrupt the flow of their thought processes. The Validation worker has to learn to converse about people or objects without being sure who, or what, they are talking about. The third hint is to use the preferred sense (stages one, two and three). This is the idea, apparently derived from Neuro-Linguistic Programming, that individuals each have a preferred sense — visual, auditory or kinaesthetic — which is expressed in their tendency to use seeing, hearing or feeling words and expressions. The Validation worker notes the preferred sense of each individual and uses words from the same sense to promote contact.

Validation Groupwork

Naomi Feil began her working life as a group therapist and it was groupwork which featured in her earliest articles and videos promoting the new and innovative approach that became Validation Therapy. My initial contact with Validation took place when Christine Bleathman and I received training in Validation groupwork techniques from Gemma Jones, who is herself a Validation Therapist trained by Feil.

Validation groupwork is more distinctive than its individual counterpart and it has weaker links with Feil's theoretical framework which developed after the group approach had become relatively established. With this in mind, I suspect that future generations will see Feil's contribution to the development of group therapy for people with dementia as her most lasting achievement.

In order to appreciate the scale of that achievement, it helps to recall the situation in dementia care at the time that Christine Bleathman and myself were preparing our research project into Validation groups in 1987. We were both working as nurses on the Felix Post Unit at the Maudsley Hospital in South London, an assessment unit and day hospital for older people diagnosed as having either functional or organic mental health problems. The ward was staffed by a highly motivated and well-trained multidisciplinary team with close links with the Section of Old Age Psychiatry at the Institute of Psychiatry, where Gemma Jones was engaged in research. While in the planning stage of our research we could not avoid sharing some of the scepticism of our nursing, medical, occupational therapist and psychologist colleagues at Gemma's insistence that a group of severely disorientated people could actively participate in therapeutic groupwork for upwards of 45 minutes at a time. Surely they would not be able to concentrate for that long? We anticipated chaotic scenes, with group members repeatedly becoming distracted, wandering about the room, calling out and interrupting each other — as people with these levels of impairment would tend to do during the RO and reminiscence sessions that were run on the ward.

My scepticism was not diminished when we recruited group members from a local Social Services Residential Home. Six people were selected initially, each being grossly disorientated in both time and place. Before any groupwork began, we spent one hour each week (for a ten-week period) observing each group member as they were in the home. We recorded all interpersonal contact in order to produce baseline measurements for our study. This process brought us face-to-face with the social void, the scarcity of psychological contact, that can pervade the daily life of residents. Each person took part in only the briefest moments of human contact, spending enormous amounts of time either alone in their rooms or, more commonly, socially isolated in a room full of people with whom they had only the most cursory of superficial interactions. The television drowned out the silence, its endless blare listened to by no-one.

The contrast between the behaviour of these cognitively impaired people in the home and how, after the group became established, they functioned in the Validation group could not have been more marked. I was astonished at the degree to which group members would remain attentive, listen to each other, follow a consistent theme and even make occasional facilitative comments in a warm, supportive and mutually encouraging atmosphere. Latent social skills were activated and used in a way that revealed the true extent of an avoidable tragedy: how the social psychology of the institution was disabling its confused residents by failing to provide an environment in which they could maintain their status as social beings. I also came to acknowledge that the creation of a prosthetic social environment could make therapeutic groupwork attainable for people who have a far greater degree of cognitive impairment than I had previously thought.

Selecting group members

In selecting group members we did not attempt to categorise residents according to the Four Stages of Disorientation, preferring to screen on the basis of their performance on the CAPE 12-item Information and Orientation Scale (Pattie & Gilleard, 1979). Members were admitted only if they scored six or less, which usually meant they were unable to identify their age, the day, month or year, or where they were. All would have been identified as being in stage two, time confusion, of the Four Stages of Resolution. They ranged from 79 to 89 years of age.

Feil recommends taking into account detailed considerations of the mix of levels of disorientation, personal qualities and other factors when forming a group and she also recommends gathering a great deal of information (as with individual Validation) on the psychosocial development of each group member (Feil, 1992a, pp83–84). As is often the case, this degree of information was simply unavailable but we did find that it was amply compensated for once the groups started, as each member gradually revealed the life events and past relationships that remained 'live' emotional issues for them. Feil also advises against including people who have a history of disruptive behaviour, but we did have one group member who was reported as having periodic outbursts of verbal aggression and physical violence towards property. This behaviour never surfaced in the group setting.

With hindsight, I suspect that much of the success of the groups was attributable to the detailed attention paid to their structure and to the physical environment in which they took place. The intention was to create an atmosphere which maximised stability, reducing to a minimum any environmental inconsistencies between meetings. This consistency was an important contributor to the development of group cohesion, as the elimination of unpredictable aspects enhanced the opportunity to focus on the content and processes in the group. It also appeared to allow group members to develop a sense of familiarity with the setting, despite only entering that room once a week for a one-hour period. The journey from the main lounge involved going up in a lift and walking along a long corridor. I remember walking to the room with Win who, despite my reassurances, clearly remained unsure as to who I was and appeared unfamiliar with the lift and the corridor. She walked tentatively, her face betraying apprehension, until the moment we entered the door of the room whereupon she visibly relaxed, announced 'Ah, we're here!', made her way over to her regular chair, sat down, smiled and assumed an expression of eager anticipation.

Such apparent familiarity is, of course, difficult to reconcile with the pronounced decrements in memory and orientation that were indicated by group members' scores on the CAPE tests. As no attempt was made to operationalise this phenomena, we have to concede that the familiarity may have been merely apparent, that group members were picking up on non-verbal cues which reflected our own increasing sense of familiarity with the group and the environment. Another possibility is that the CAPE scores were artificially low, perhaps indicating an under-performance for which environmental and affective factors were partially responsible. We must also, however, keep in mind evidence (for example, Godden & Baddeley, 1975) which suggests that recall is improved by subjects being in the same environmental context in which information was originally learnt. Similarly, the consistency of ambience from group to group may have contributed to an affective consistency in group members which assisted memory function. It is known that mood has a strong 'context effect' on memory, with studies showing that information learnt when sad, for example, is best recalled when sad (for example, Bower, 1981).

Five-Minute Warning

The groups were held every Wednesday morning at 11am, at which time functioning was, we were assured, at its height. Some five to ten minutes before the group began, the group workers would locate each of the group members in the home, introduce themselves and remind them that they would shortly return to accompany them to 'the meeting'. We would often be greeted at this stage by a polite, if embarrassed, puzzlement, the meetings being held weekly and our faces unrecognised after seven days' absence. It did mean, however, that when we reappeared to escort them to the group a few minutes later our faces might seem a little less unfamiliar and group members had some chance to adjust to the idea that they were about to be going somewhere.

Physical Environment

There were usually seven to eight people in each group (five or six members and two staff). The appropriate number of comfortable chairs were pre-arranged in a circle, close enough for each person to hold the hand of the person on either side. Group members always sat in the same seat, as did the two group workers who sat opposite each other. A room was selected on the basis that it comfortably held this number of chairs but was not so large as to prevent the development of an intimate, 'cosy' atmosphere.

The Group Songs

One consistent feature was the group songs with which we would open and close the sessions. Our group chose 'When You're Smiling' as the opening song and 'Side-by-Side' to close with. Given that group members with this level of impairment generally find singing familiar songs less challenging than speaking, starting with a song allows everybody to vocalise early in the group in the hope that this will build confidence for active participation.

Group Roles

Our group songs were started off by Betty, who became established as our 'songleader'. Each group member would take on a role within the group, which conferred some status on them. In this group the four members who attended most regularly took on roles of songleader, welcomer, thanker and hostess. Naomi Feil suggests that group roles should be allocated in advance, based on the likelihood of group members preferring one particular role to another (Feil, 1992a, p84). We were more comfortable with the idea of allowing two or three sessions in which group members would be encouraged to try out the different roles before settling on one which they felt most suited to.

It is preferable to have two group workers and a maximum of eight group members (Feil suggests five to ten), with one of the group workers acting as a lead worker and the other as a support. The lead worker is responsible for moving the group on through the protocol, inviting contributions from all group members, drawing together themes and shared conclusions and making appropriate process comments. The support worker sits opposite the lead worker, so as to be aware of the group members on either side of the lead worker. Their role is to deal with any practical assistance that may be required with toiletting and so on and also to pick up on the reactions of individual group members that the leader may miss.

Starting the Group

Once everybody was seated the group leader would stand and go around each person in the group, shaking them by the hand and thanking them for coming. The group leader would then invite the welcomer to say a few words of greeting, after which the songleader would be asked to start us off on the opening song.

The Content of the Groups

The two group workers would agree with the project supervisor potential themes and topics, selected on the basis that they either broached new areas or expanded on themes that had already arisen. These would usually form a contingency plan as, after the initial few groups, it was more common for a theme to arise spontaneously and for the content to be driven by the group members themselves. A lot of the discussion was around personalised reminiscences — about parents, siblings, partners, children, special occasions — but more current issues, such as what it is like to live in a home, how it feels to grow old, problems with memory and attitudes to death, were also dealt with.

Despite the apparent cognitive deficits revealed by the CAPE assessments, group members were able to remain focused on a particular theme or topic for much longer periods than had appeared possible outside of the group. This was probably a result of the very direct attempts of the group workers to involve each member of the group in the discussion from the outset. As a topic of conversation arose, the group worker would directly address those members who had not spoken and ask for their views and thoughts. Similarly, any member who had not spoken for some time, or who appeared to be losing concentration, would be given a brief summary of the point that had been reached and invited to contribute. This constant vigilance by the group workers helped group members remain engaged in conversations for longer than would ordinarily be possible, a fact appreciated by Edith in the extract below, despite her inability to recall the frequency of meetings.

Edith:	Oh I'm pleased to be here. Especially now I've got into the meetings and I see Reg, although I see him all the week, you can't have much of a conversation, can you?
Reg:	No.
Edith:	But when we meet once a day, once a week, whatever it is, I think that's lovely, I really do.
Reg:	Brings you more together
Edith:	Definitely, yes, you know what each other wants, unhappiness and happiness.

(Bleathman & Morton, 1992, p661)

Whilst none of our group's members suffered from any significant degree of dysphasia, the degree of their disorientation would fluctuate. The following extract shows how factually inaccurate comments (Edith was not getting married and Win was, in fact, alone) did not significantly disrupt the flow of the conversation or the feelings being expressed.

Edith:	I'm going to get married again and I hope you'll all come to the wedding because I know I'm going to be very happy.
Groupworker:	You'd like to get married again would you Edith?
Edith:	I can't bear to think of living alone.
Groupworker:	Do you feel like you live alone here?
Edith:	Oh yes, all alone.
Reg:	Get it off your chest a little bit and then you'll feel a lot better.
Edith:	Yes, I feel like you're one of me.
Reg:	Otherwise it stops it building up.
Edith: (to Win)	Would you get married again?
Win:	I think so, yes, but I'm not alone.
Edith:	You're not. Oh.
Win:	No. I'm thinking how I would feel if I were.

| Groupworker: | You were putting yourself in Edith's shoes. |
| Edith: | It's not very nice to be alone. |

(Bleathman & Morton, 1992, p663)

Ending the Group

The group leader invariably had the task of winding up the group's discussion as the time approached for the group to finish. At a suitable moment, the leader would interject, thanking whoever had been speaking for their contribution and, if appropriate, suggest that the subject be picked up again at the following week's meeting. The songleader would then be invited to start the closing song before the meeting was formally closed by the thanker. After the group had finished, the host/ess would be assisted by the support worker in passing round the soft drinks and biscuits prior to the group members being helped to return to the home's main lounge.

Reflections and Comments on Validation Practice

Any evaluation of the practice of Validation should acknowledge Feil's insistence that it ought to be judged by the quality of the relationship that is established between the therapist and the disorientated person. The attitude, personal qualities and interpersonal skill the therapist brings to the relationship will be more important than any techniques that they use in determining the success of any intervention.

In making this point, Feil echoes that made by Rogers (1957b) when he argued that the therapeutic relationship is essential to any positive personality change. This notion leaves considerable difficulties for researchers as the quality of any human relationship is, while recognisable, notoriously troublesome to measure. Nonetheless, Feil is obviously correct to warn against the temptation to use the techniques of Validation in a mechanistic and disinterested way. These techniques should be seen as guides as to possibilities, rather than prescriptions without alternatives.

That having been said, there are a few areas where the guidance Feil offers is, I believe, questionable. One such instance arises from the examples of interactions with people who are said to be in stage three, repetitive motion. This group is distinguished by having marked expressive dysphasia which has left them unable to utilise language to communicate effectively. In Feil's words, they 'communicate mainly on a non-verbal level [and] substitute movement for speech' (Feil, 1992a, p109). This group is, therefore, very vulnerable to having their actions interpreted on the basis of the 'theory of symbols' which has been discussed above. My specific objection is that many examples of Validation interactions which are modelled in the literature show the results of Feil's conviction that disorientated people are returning to the past, perhaps to a time when they felt useful, perhaps to a time of particular crisis. In either event, the result reads rather like a game of charades, or perhaps like the panel game, 'What's my Line?', where contestants are asked to guess the occupation being mimed. We see something of this in the example in van Amelsvoort Jones (1985) above and also in this extract from Feil:

> A purse symbolizes a filing cabinet for a former file-clerk. She files, filling her purse with Kleenex. The Kleenex becomes the vital documents she folded as a legal secretary. Another woman uses her purse as an oven. She was a housewife, giving her family joy by baking bread. She pats, placing the dough in the oven, restoring her feelings of dignity and motherhood.
> (Feil, 1982, p42)

I do question the wisdom of arriving at any interaction with individuals who have been identified (even labelled?) as being in stage three with the preconceived idea that their behaviour is likely be a re-enactment of some scene or situation from their earlier lives. Feil confidently asserts that the person in stage three will let us know when we make the wrong interpretation, but does not provide us with any evidence on which such confidence might be based. Given that expressive dysphasia is likely to be accompanied by a significant degree of receptive dysphasia, there is a reasonable chance that the person in stage three may not even be in a position to understand our interpretation of their behaviour. Clearly, then, they will not be in a position to correct any misinterpretation we may make.

Regarding group Validation, Feil has clearly made an important contribution to the development of our ability to engage people with a moderate degree of dementia in therapeutic groupwork. In using the term 'therapeutic', I mean groupwork that assists individuals by sharing, and coming to terms with, personally significant, emotionally laden, material through a group process which is dependent upon the creation of a supportive and psychologically safe environment. Feil was the first person to seriously contemplate this kind of approach to people with dementia, and the eclectic range of contributors to her theoretical base is reflected in the development of Validation groups. Much of the content of Validation groupwork consists of 'life review' reminiscence work, as inspired by Butler (1963), facilitated by workers employing standard groupwork techniques, or dealing with more 'here and now' concerns with a Rogerian emphasis. The structure of the groups — the protocol and group members' roles — appears to have a further enabling effect and Feil's assembling of these various components was an important step in the advance of dementia care. In the future, however, I suspect that the lack of substance, cohesion and unity in Feil's theoretical frame will leave practitioners feeling at liberty to select and use those aspects of her practice that they feel to be potentially useful, and to disregard the rest. Whilst this would lead to the eventual demise of Validation Therapy as such, it would not undermine either the influence it has had or its historical significance.

CHAPTER 3

Resolution Therapy

A TWENTY-YEAR PERIOD elapsed between the appearance of Naomi Feil's earliest published article in the United States (Feil, 1967) and the first signs that her ideas were beginning to gain some influence in Britain (Morton & Bleathman, 1988). Only in the latter half of the 1980s did the culture of dementia care in this country begin to show signs of a serious interest in the emotional world of the dementia sufferer. Growing alongside this interest was an acceptance of the possibility that psychological approaches could address that inner emotional world. Reality Orientation (RO), which had continued to dominate, was being increasingly discredited in the eyes of many caregivers, especially as it was widely practised in a mechanistic manner. It had come to be seen as dismissive of the emotions and perceptions of people with dementia. The enormous interest provoked by the initial appearance of Validation was indicative of how ill-equipped caregivers had come to feel when faced with the human needs of someone with dementia.

Resolution Therapy, the product of a collaboration between Fiona Goudie and Graham Stokes, attracted a similar degree of attention on the basis of just one short article (Goudie & Stokes, 1989) and one chapter in a book (Stokes & Goudie, 1990). It represents the first British attempt to meet the growing demand from caregivers requiring assistance in meeting the emotional needs of people with dementia.

Background

Goudie and Stokes, both clinical psychologists, began working together in the mid-1980s in Coventry. Goudie was at this time working in the community settings, which brought her into contact with a number of older clients in the (sometimes undiagnosed) earlier stages of a dementing illness. As she was already utilising the same therapeutic skills with these people that she would use with cognitively intact older people, she began to question why professionals were not motivated to build a therapeutic alliance — based on acceptance, congruence and empathy and using active and reflective listening skills — with distressed older people with dementia, as they would be with older people who were diagnosed as suffering from depression, or from anxiety. Graham Stokes had already published a series of short guides to managing some of the common behavioural problems shown by people with dementia. His approach combined the use of problem-solving techniques developed by behaviour modification with a concern to understand behaviour in the context of the individual's attempt to make sense of, adapt to and react to their environment. He stressed that difficult behaviour can often best be dealt with by modifying environments that fail to meet psychological needs.

In 1987, Goudie and Stokes established a five-day training course entitled 'Working with Dementia', which was later to become the title of the book they edited. They ran the course, which incorporated a wide range of psychological approaches to working with confused older people, in a variety of places throughout Britain, attracting large numbers of participants. It became clear that their students, largely trained nurses, occupational therapists and social workers, showed far more interest in the emotional world of the dementia sufferer than previous generations of these professions had done. An awareness of the need for the course to address these issues, and their contact with Una Holden, stimulated Goudie and Stokes to examine the early literature on Reality Orientation. Whilst they acknowledged that 'RO is not simply a mechanistic technique to improve retention of information' (Goudie & Stokes, 1989, p35), they did feel that RO actually had aims other than meeting the affective needs of people with dementia.

They were enthusiastic about their first contact with Validation but had concerns that Validation did not go far enough: that if people were expressing feelings resulting from depression, or from anxiety, it was not enough simply to validate that expression — an attempt needed to be made to deal with the source of the distress, to resolve the issue. We might say that whereas, for Goudie and Stokes, resolution would indicate necessary modifications to the environment, Validation, for Feil, was the necessary modification to the environment.

Goudie and Stokes also felt that Feil's insistence that the distress of disorientated older people was likely to involve an attempt to deal with conflicts from the past could divert staff from possible causes of distress in the 'here and now'. They cautioned against the dangers of a psychodynamic interpretation of confused speech and behaviour as:

It deflects staff from the probable underlying content and feelings which are masked by the confused message. Second, it inappropriately attributes the dementia sufferer with the intellectual and analytical powers necessary for abstract reasoning, fantasy development and the use of defence mechanism when confronted with distressing emotions which deteriorate markedly as the disease progresses.

(Ibid., pp36–37)

Feeling that neither RO nor Validation was able to fill the vacuum of therapeutic approaches, Goudie and Stokes began to look at the skills they had been trained to use with people diagnosed as suffering from a functional mental illness. It was their discussions around the applicability of such skills and techniques to dementia that led them to be amongst the first published advocates of a position that has since gained such widespread acceptance that it now appears quite unremarkable. The position can be summarised as the following propositions:

1 that people with an organic mental health problem can, and often do, also have a degree of affective disorder; and

2 that there is no fundamental reason why such disorders in people with a dementia should not respond to the same types of psychological intervention that are used with people who do not have a dementia.

Thus, whilst Goudie and Stokes do not question the classificatory division of psychiatric disorders into organic and functional illnesses, they do challenge a set of assumptions about the implications of that division. These assumptions, widespread at the end of the 1980s, had led them to the development of one set of psychological approaches for people with functional illnesses and another set for people with dementia, almost as if the latter were losing not only their cognitive powers but also their capacity to experience, and to feel, as human beings.

Like Validation, Resolution Therapy entails paying close attention to all attempted communication by people with dementia. Whereas Feil believes confused speech and behaviour is probably understandable in psychodynamic terms, Goudie and Stokes, however, argued that it is more likely to be either an attempt at communicating expressions of current need or an effort to make sense of the environment. They view dementia as a barrier to communication and contact, referring to a 'struggle to negotiate and make sense of reality through a mist of confusion' (Stokes & Goudie, 1990, p185). The task of Resolution Therapy was to overcome that barrier: 'By using the counselling skills of reflective listening, exploration, warmth and acceptance in the Rogerian "reflection of feelings" tradition, nurses can empathise with the hidden meaning and feelings which lie behind confused verbal and behavioural expressions' (Goudie & Stokes, 1989, p37).

Confused speech or behaviour is seen as an attempt at communication. In order to respond the caregiver attempts to discern the meaning concealed by the confusion, by making a tentative attempt to identify and acknowledge the feeling that may accompany the message. If so indicated, there may need to be practical changes to meet the needs that have been made known, as in the example below.

Setting:	Confused man sitting in a day-room. Other patients sitting in armchairs. Room is of a 'waiting-room' design. TV is on.

Confused message: behaviour:	He starts to move furniture around the room, resisting staff efforts to get him to sit down.
Concealed meaning:	I am bored. I need to be active. I need to feel useful.
Underlying feelings:	Boredom. Irritation. Discontent.
Reflective response:	It gets boring just sitting around sometimes, doesn't it? Is there anything you'd like to do?
Resolution:	Once an attempt is made to understand the person's feelings, practical attempts such as modifying their environment or providing a choice of activities will enhance acknowledgement and help the patient to work through or resolve the expression of their feelings. (Adapted from Stokes & Goudie, 1990, pp184–188)

Whilst Goudie and Stokes clearly believe that psychosocial interventions can produce benefits to affect and behaviour, they also accept the inevitability of the disease progressing to a stage when the barrier to further communication and contact will become insurmountable. In the meantime, however, they suggest that, by adapting the use of Rogerian reflective counselling skills, we can be assisted in understanding confused expressions of need. It is hoped that such contact will alleviate the sense of isolation and also point to possible modifications in the physical environment, or in the psychosocial milieu, which will remove sources of distress. Such techniques are to be used until there are objective signs that distress has diminished. The need for frequent 'repeat doses', as memory problems will ensure that many of the gains that are made will be short-lived, means that Resolution Therapy is most effective when employed by those carers who are in regular and frequent contact with the person with dementia.

Reflections and Comments
It is perhaps more appropriate to consider resolution less as a 'therapy' in its own right and more as an invocation to adapt Rogerian

counselling skills to assist with 'understanding and acknowledging the current feelings of the confused individual ... finding ways to help the person cope with these feelings ... [which may include] ... modifications to the environment and nurse–patient relationships' (Goudie & Stokes, 1989, p37).

In other words, it emphasised that the confused articulations and behaviour of people with dementia are likely to be about something, and that if we learn to listen we may well be able to work out what the meaning is and, if necessary, act to improve the situation. It may seem strange now that such a statement was ever necessary, as it has become one of the foundations of the 'new culture of dementia care', but perhaps this is an indication of the extent of the ground that resolution and its successors gained in the field of person-centred dementia care.

The fact that only a couple of introductory articles were published, however, leaves us with a number of unanswered questions about the application of Rogerian principles to dementia care. Many of these have been picked up by Tom Kitwood and his colleagues in Bradford but a logical next step for Goudie and Stokes to have followed would have been an examination of the nature of the therapeutic relationship involving someone who has a dementia. For Rogers, the end result of showing the 'core conditions', and of using reflective practice, is the development of a therapeutic relationship that becomes the 'vehicle' of therapeutic movement, insight or change. Whilst we might have more modest ambitions when working with someone who has a dementia, we might justifiably argue that enhancing the potential to make and maintain close, good quality personal relationships would be a very worthwhile goal for dementia care. In order to make progress in this area, we would need to consider the extent to which the formation of relationships is dependent upon cognitive factors, in order to identify areas in which compensatory strategies would need to developed.

This question is obviously more complex than it first appears. Trust, for example, would tend to be in most people's lists of the necessary ingredients for a good quality relationship and we tend to think of trust as being something that is learnt on a case-by-case basis: I learn to trust A because A repeatedly demonstrates good intentions towards me whereas I learn not to trust B because B is erratic in this regard. The problem, however, is that many people with severe memory impairment and difficulties with retention appear to build relationships that involve a degree of trust. I am often struck by the way some of the people with dementia who attend the day centre at which I work appear to form a set of relationships — with staff members and with other attendees — which are remarkably consistent from week to week, even though they may attend on just one day each week. On arrival, if tested, they may be able to provide no evidence to indicate they remember having attended before, yet, on an interpersonal level, they pick up more or less where they left off the previous week.

Aside from this obvious criticism of its incomplete nature, there are two further comments on Resolution Therapy that are worth making. The first point concerns the strength of the emphasis that confused speech and behaviour is likely to reflect about the 'here and now' reality of the person with dementia. Whilst this point was obviously made as a contrast to the psychodynamic interpretations of Validation, it is a point that is made too strongly. The reality is that people with dementia do often sometimes behave as if they are back in some earlier part of their lives, and that when they do so their emotional responses can only be understood by reference to the situation that they perceive themselves to be in. Equally, it is true to say that, sometimes, confused speech and behaviour represents concerns with the here and now, or an attempt to make sense of their current environment. The point is that it is unhelpful to enter any interaction carrying preconceptions about the nature of the content that the person with dementia will be trying to communicate. The less we assume, the better we will listen.

Finally, I should point out that the article on resolution is perhaps too pessimistic about the possibility of keeping meaningful communication alive, at least until the very late stages of a dementia: 'We, of course, accept that as the dementia progresses, opportunities for counselling or work on acknowledging feelings diminishes' (Goudie & Stokes, 1989, p37). Although increasing language difficulties will undoubtedly lessen the opportunities for verbal counselling, there is ample evidence to suggest that the barriers to non-verbal communication will continue to be surmountable long after this point has been reached. Our acknowledgement of the way that another person is feeling is carried out in a language that is very largely non-verbal, hardly surprising when we consider that it is a language that we learn in the first weeks of life, well before we are able to speak or to understand a word. Fiona Goudie, in her work with stroke victims with impoverished verbal skills, now argues that much work on emotional distress can be done non-verbally, through the use of reflective skills such as those of mirroring. Nor should we ever underestimate the communicative power of touch, facial expression, voice tone and other cues through which we can gain a more accurate perception of the levels of another's acceptance, congruence and empathy than we ever could from the words that they speak.

Whilst there may be few caregivers today who would describe themselves as 'resolution therapists', I believe it would be a mistake to underestimate the significance of Goudie and Stokes' contribution to the development of person-centred dementia care. When they argued that people with dementia are subject to similar emotional processes, amenable to similar interventions to those experienced by anybody else, they brought the dementia sufferer right back into the world of persons. In this they were succeeded by another British psychologist, Tom Kitwood, and his colleagues at the Bradford Dementia Group.

CHAPTER 4

Tom Kitwood, the Bradford Dementia Group and Spring Mount

Introduction: from 'Therapies' to 'Approaches to Care'

The extent of the interest which greeted the appearance of Resolution Therapy was indicative of the growth of confidence in the possibility of developing psychotherapeutic approaches to the care of people suffering from dementia. Its founders were well aware, however, of the need to modify the conventional practices of psychotherapy if resolution was to benefit individuals suffering from increasing cognitive deficits. Any progress made in the traditional weekly or fortnightly session would prove increasingly short-lived in the face of advancing memory impairment. The 'therapy' was, therefore, particularly ill-suited to being ' ... conducted at certain times of the day in a formal setting' (Goudie & Stokes, 1989, p37). To be effective, Goudie and Stokes argued, resolution needs to be practised at every appropriate opportunity by those who are in most frequent contact with the person with dementia. Hence the fact that, although written by a pair of clinical psychologists, the one published article on resolution appeared in a popular nursing journal, on the grounds that 'Nurses are in daily contact and communication with dementing patients and, therefore, have an enormous therapeutic potential for this approach' (ibid.).

This ambition, for resolution to become a characteristic feature of the care milieu, perhaps calls into question the appropriateness of its being described as a 'therapy' — a suggestion that has echoes in debates taking place elsewhere. Supporters of Validation, for example, have addressed similar issues surrounding the use of the term 'therapy', which carries different meanings on either side of the North Atlantic. In Europe, the term 'therapy' is usually taken to carry the same meaning as 'treatment'. It commonly refers to a defined physical or psychological intervention, occurring over a discrete period of time and, more often than not, carried out by a trained, qualified, practitioner. In North American usage, however, 'therapy' has less precise connotations, tending to describe anything that is designed to help a person. Thus, whilst Validation groups might be said to meet the European definition of therapy, it appears that individual Validation — in view of its continuous nature — might be more appropriately described in Europe as an 'approach' or 'method'.

Similar points could be made in relation to Reality Orientation (in its '24 hour' form) and to Resolution. Indeed, there are good reasons to suggest that the process of losing our mental powers to dementia is such that we are always more likely to be helped by approaches that are continuous, and that we are always better advised to think in terms of 'approaches to care' and 'psychological environments' than 'treatments' or 'interventions'. The early 1990s saw a growing consensus around this view, emphasising the therapeutic potential, and status, of care. Such a consensus was evidenced by the publication of titles such as *Care-Giving in Dementia* (Jones & Miesen) in 1992 and the appearance of the influential *Journal of Dementia Care* in the following year. It was to find its most articulate theoretician and exponent in the psychologist Tom Kitwood, who came to the field of dementia having previously specialised in the psychology of conscience, of moral development and of caring.

Kitwood's Background

Kitwood's distinctive, even radical, approach to dementia is in part explained by his having arrived at the subject via a very different route from that taken by most of his peers. Whereas the majority of psychologists working with dementia have received a training in clinical psychology, Kitwood's professional background lay in psychotherapy and counselling, including a training in Gestalt. As a medical student he had studied some neuroscience and he followed this by studying social psychology, being strongly influenced by the ethogenics of Rom Harré. This background provided him with a relatively diverse, yet relevant, set of perspectives, each of which played their part in the development of an account of dementia which has a breadth surpassing anything yet produced by his contemporaries. It is an account that has certainly captured the imagination of a large and influential section of those involved in dementia care.

A retrospective review of Kitwood's publications on dementia reveals a strikingly logical progression to his work. In his earliest articles the central theme is the 'medicalisation' of dementia — an almost social constructionist account of the creation of the accepted wisdom that dementia is a purely organic mental illness. Having described the triumph of what he calls the 'standard paradigm' view of dementia, Kitwood moved on to a critique of the empirical evidence and the philosophical foundations which support it. Finding these to be lacking, he then developed an alternative conceptual framework which employed ideas and constructs derived from social psychology and psychotherapy. This in turn led him to identify significant non-biological influences in dementia (the 'Malignant Social Psychology') which he sought to quantify and influence by developing the evaluative tool of Dementia Care Mapping. More recently, his work involved a shift in focus away from the negative effects of bad care towards the positive effects of good care, a concerted effort to understand good practice and how it might be promoted. Through all these phases he collaborated with a number of colleagues, most notably those from the Bradford Dementia Group (formerly the Bradford Dementia Research Group) which has, under Kitwood's direction, emerged to become one of the most influential and progressive forces in dementia care today.

The Medicalisation of Alzheimer's Disease

There are comparisons to be drawn between Kitwood's early work on dementia and that of authors such as R.D. Laing and David Cooper, who led the 'anti-psychiatry' movement of the 1960s and 1970s. For Kitwood's project also involved a direct challenge to the hegemony of the medical perspective on mental health problems, locating the 'medicalisation' of dementia as a characteristic feature of the power relationships predominating in 'late capitalist' or 'modern industrial' societies.

Indeed, a casual reader of Kitwood's earliest published article on dementia could be forgiven for concluding that Kitwood is denying the existence of any pathological element in Alzheimer's Disease at all, particularly when he writes: 'how much social construction is involved in rendering Alzheimer's as a disease entity' (Kitwood, 1987a, p82) and then reports approvingly Gubrium and Lynnott's (1985) view that ''Alzheimer's Disease' is little more than an acceptable new code for giving meaning to some of the troubles which typically arise in late life' (Kitwood, 1987a, p82), a code that, in Kitwood's view, 'resonates with some of our most endemic forms of alienation' (ibid.).

Later articles (for example, Kitwood, 1990a) make it clear, however, that Kitwood did acknowledge the existence of a genuine neuropathology at work in dementia. His opposition was to the almost total exclusion of other factors and perspectives which could, he held, enhance both our understanding of the causal processes in dementia and our ability to mitigate its effects. This exclusion is explained in the early writings in terms of the origins, growth and nature of the ideology attached to what he would later describe as the 'old culture' of dementia care. It was an ideology that had emerged triumphant as the 'standard paradigm' view which sought to explain dementia purely in terms of the progress of a neuropathology.

Kitwood saw that the standard paradigm account of dementia is an example of the biological reductionism which continues to hold influence in western psychiatry, despite now appearing quite extreme when considered on its own merits. This reductionism rests on two complementary premises:

1 that all descriptions of mental processes — thoughts, beliefs, feelings, perceptions and so on — can ultimately be reduced (in theory at least) to descriptions of the physical, biochemical processes occurring in the brain/nervous system; and
2 that descriptions of the physical processes taking place in the brain/nervous system have, intrinsically, greater explanatory power than descriptions which employ constructs such as 'thoughts', 'beliefs', 'feelings', 'perceptions' and so on which are neither observable nor measurable.

One implication of this position is that everything learnt from psychology could, in principle at least, be learnt from physiology which in turn implies that the supremacy of natural science is such that one day we may expect the former to be replaced by the latter. In the philosophy of science, it is a view closely associated with the logical positivist movement of the inter-war years. At a time when the intellectual prestige associated with the natural sciences was at its height, the positivists advocated the application of 'scientific' principles and methods to other areas of human thought. They argued that in order to speak meaningfully, in any context, it is necessary to make statements that are empirically verifiable and, whilst their influence waned as awareness of Einsteinian physics (which employed concepts that were not empirically verifiable) grew, much of the dominant 'medical model' in western psychiatry continued to develop in the direction that positivism had set.

In relation to dementia, the absolute identification of 'mind' and 'brain' implied by the standard paradigm entails that our attempt to understand the actions and experiences of any person with dementia need involve us looking no further than to the effects of neuropathology and to the resultant damage to cognitions. As a consequence of this identification, Kitwood complained, dementia 'stands out as having been virtually untouched by psychoanalysis and its derivatives' (Kitwood, 1987b, p117).

That this was not always the case is shown by Kitwood being able to point to a number of authors, writing between 1925 and 1975, who took a somewhat more holistic view of the causes of dementia. They developed hypotheses based on an interaction of the psychological and the neuropathological. Only since the publication of some key research studies in the 1970s, Kitwood maintained, has the full weight of medicotechnical opinion prevailed, allowing the standard paradigm view to make an almost exclusive claim to being the orthodox, 'commonsense', view of dementia. Chief amongst its casualties were explanations of dementia which sought to incorporate psychological and social factors which were becoming disregarded in research and overlooked as possible contributors to individual cases.

Whilst the research studies of the 1970s may have provided some rationale, however questionable, for the acceptance of the standard paradigm, they do not provide a sufficient explanation of its triumph. Other factors were also at work, not least the compatibility of the standard paradigm view with the influential 'medical model' account of mental health problems in general. Explanations of mental health problems which cast them as diseases affecting certain unfortunate individuals, in which the central dynamic is played out between the disease process and the individual, continue to flourish. They accord with the individualised perspective of health problems that remains a characteristic of the western medical tradition, alongside its tendency to rely exclusively on the kinds of understanding that are provided by the natural sciences. They stand in sharp contrast to the standpoint that Kitwood adopted, maintaining that the psychological problems of any individual can only be understood with reference to their own unique biography, a biography that can itself only be understood in the context of the social relations in which it unfolds (Kitwood, 1987a, p84). In general, however, the understanding offered by psychology and the social sciences has continually been underplayed: 'At least since the time of Rudolf Virchow in the nineteenth century, medicine in the West has been tending to deal with human ill-being not primarily through an engagement with persons but through an inquiry into the pathological process in organs and cells' (Kitwood, 1987b, p134). The prevalence of this mode of engagement amongst successive generations of the medical community left the majority of its members bereft of the 'skills of interpersonal understanding, which require a person to have a well-developed awareness and tolerance of his or her own subjectivity' (ibid., p135).

In the light of the medical profession's collective lack of awareness of intellectual life beyond the horizons of the natural sciences, we should not be surprised, Kitwood suggested, that research programmes into dementia have focused almost exclusively upon investigations of neuropathology. The central assumption behind the standard paradigm — that dementia is a purely neuropathological process — has been accepted before work on the design of research programmes has even begun.

The influence exerted by the medical profession over other health professionals ensured that this position remained hegemonic. Nursing remains ideologically subservient to medicine, as is demonstrated by its passive acceptance of the medical view of dementia (ibid.), and the continuing preoccupation of clinical psychology with cognitive functioning (Kitwood & Bredin, 1992a, p278) is testament to its failure to develop a distinct conceptualisation and approach. We might also make the point, in addition to Kitwood's observations, that the somewhat dismissive attitude that Freud and many of his successors held towards the potential use of psychoanalysis and its derivatives with older people (without even considering those with dementia) has itself hindered the development of an alternative to the medical view.

Such is the scale of public prestige accorded to medical opinion that we might have expected carers and other members of the public to accept the standard paradigm, even before they were tempted to collude with its assumptions by the psychological comforts that Kitwood believed it supplies. He pointed out how the presumption that life events and the psychological environment play a contributory role in the genesis and course of a dementia can threaten to implicate relatives and other carers. Thus the guilt that carers habitually experience leaves them all the more ready to accept the fatalistic consolation of believing that they themselves could not possibly be a factor in the decline that they witness. The idea of a remorseless, progressive neuropathology enables family carers to avoid having to face up to the possibility of their own involvement — past, present and future — in the fate of the person with dementia. Kitwood was realistic enough to recognise that this avoidance is, in many cases, absolutely essential if carers are not to become totally overwhelmed by the extent of the physical and emotional demands that are placed upon them.

Whatever comfort the standard paradigm view of dementia may offer to carers is more than outweighed by the damage that Kitwood saw resulting from its acceptance. We have been persuaded, *en masse*, to take a step back and adopt a technical understanding of the 'psychic disintegration' (Kitwood, 1987a, p82) of our fellow human beings. Such is the effect of diagnosing any individual as having a 'disease' which, it is believed, will largely determine their future psychological state. It persuades those around them that the quality of their social and interpersonal life will now play little or no part in their future psychological well-being. This has obvious and profound repercussions for the way the person with dementia is treated by others, often, in Kitwood's view, serving as a further justification for carers avoiding a: 'serious engagement with the subjectivity of confused old people' (Kitwood, 1987b, p137).

Such a lack of engagement would be thought of as inexcusable in relation to someone with a mental health problem that is perceived as being comprehensible in psychotherapeutic terms. It is characteristic, however, of the 'old culture of dementia care' and of the standard paradigm view which, at best, condemns both sufferers and caregivers to adopting a passive role in relation to dementia, with the caregiver restricted to administering palliative care as the remorseless disease process takes its inevitable toll.

It was these apparent connections between the way that people with dementia are treated and the way that dementia is understood that convinced Kitwood of the need to re-examine the way we think about dementia. The 'neuropathic ideology' (Kitwood, 1997a, p36) was not just mistaken, it was actually doing great harm. The reconceptualisation of dementia was, therefore, no mere academic exercise, it was driven by a moral imperative to improve the lot of real, suffering, human beings.

Kitwood's Critique of the Standard Paradigm

Any serious challenge to the dominance of the 'medical model' of dementia must do more than account for its origins, ascendancy and place in the sociopolitical order. It must also confront the arguments used to support the orthodox position and present a credible alternative. Kitwood included both a sustained critique of the standard paradigm and a persuasive attempt to reconceptualise dementia by utilising concepts from social psychology and from the various psychotherapeutic traditions.

We have seen that the standard paradigm, in Kitwood's analysis, constitutes the central theoretical pillar supporting the classification of dementia as a purely 'organic' mental illness. As such, it is primarily a causal explanation, maintaining that there are disease entities (most commonly Alzheimer's and vascular diseases) which become manifested in neuropathological processes, a description of which can wholly account for the 'symptoms' we identify with dementia. Whilst the origins of the disease entity are, at present, obscure (at least in the case of Alzheimer's) it is assumed that the path to their discovery will be cleared by increasing knowledge of the relevant neurological processes. Consequently, any 'treatment' which hopes to have an impact on the course of the disease is likely to be pharmacological, designed to influence neurological processes and thus delay, arrest or even reverse the onset of symptoms. Kitwood (1989, p2) expressed the linear causal chain which underpins the paradigm as:

$$X \longrightarrow \text{neuropathic change} \longrightarrow \text{dementia}$$

Where 'X' is a one or more causal agents, currently unknown in Alzheimer's Disease but better understood in the vascular dementias.

This standard paradigm account of dementia remains instantly recognisable to professionals involved in dementia care and it forms the basis of the 'public image' of Alzheimer's Disease as an irresistibly degenerative neurological disorder. In the initial stages of his challenge to this account (Kitwood, 1987b) Kitwood conducted a critical examination of the research evidence reputed to justify the belief in an exclusive causal link between the neuropathology, on the one hand, and the dementing process, on the other. Examining in detail some of the key research studies published between 1968 and 1986, he concluded that, whilst it is undeniable that 'Underlying senile dementia there is, of course, a process of degeneration of nervous tissue' (ibid., p138), the weakness of the correlation between the observed clinical 'symptoms' displayed during life and the extent of the neurological damage revealed post-mortem indicates that the studies 'do not entail the conclusion of exclusive neuropathological causation' (ibid., p131).

In other words, there is insufficient evidence to rule out the possibility that social and psychological factors play a significant causal role in both the onset and the course of a dementing illness. Indeed, the weakness of the correlation is such that 'there is no possibility of Alzheimer's or vascular dementia meeting the key criterion of a classical disease: that distinct pathological features should be present in all cases where the symptoms appear, and in none of the cases where they do not' (Kitwood, 1997a, p25).

In addition to this critique of the research base supporting the standard paradigm, Kitwood also questioned its ability to account for some commonly witnessed features of dementia. The first relates to individuals who are diagnosed as suffering from a dementing illness as a result of developing most, if not all, of the key 'symptoms' of dementia (memory impairment, disorientation, dyspraxia, dysphasia and so on) in the absence of any 'acute' cause (infections, drug toxicity and so on) and who then either recover their cognitive abilities or are found, post-mortem, to show no evidence of neurological damage. Such cases have often been described as 'pseudo-dementia', which is held to be a functional illness (usually depression) which 'masquerades' as, or mimics, dementia. The problem with this explanation, as Kitwood points out, is that it leaves clinicians unable to make a confident diagnosis of dementia prior to death. Furthermore, the creation of the construct 'pseudo-dementia' actually undermines the causal account of dementia as it is contained in the standard paradigm. For if non-neuropathological factors can induce the same clinical symptoms as dementia during a lifetime, how are we to know that it is not similar factors that are the true cause of the same symptoms in someone who does happen to have a marked neuropathology revealed at autopsy?

Secondly, an account of dementia as a purely organic disease which develops according to its own dynamic leaves us without an explanation for the numerous anecdotal examples of the 'apparent precipitation' of dementia following major life crises, especially bereavement (Kitwood, 1989, p4). Again an 'ad hoc' standard paradigm explanation of these cases has grown up, involving the claim that the deceased partner must have been compensating for, or covering up, the bereaved person's cognitive deficits which only became apparent when they were no longer around to do so. But this explanation is too readily dismissive of the powers of observation of close family members, neighbours and others who have been in close contact with the person with dementia before and after their loss. Their accounts of a real change in the level of functioning following the loss of a spouse may lack the methodological rigour of a well designed research study, but it is often based on a good deal of very close observation and deserves to be taken seriously as a source of evidence.

The suggestion that psychological factors may have a causal role in triggering the onset of dementia has its counterpart in the view that they can also have a significant impact on the rate of increase in the severity of symptoms. Documented examples of 'catastrophic decline' in dementia sufferers following changes in their care or in their environment add to the growing evidence of a link between neuropathology and stress. Studies that suggest a relationship involving increased stress in dementia with both increased mortality (Robertson *et al*, 1993) and decreased quality of life (Bredin *et al*, 1995) have encouraged acceptance of the possibility that stress may also be linked to the rate of cognitive decline: a 'stress hypothesis' (Kitwood, 1997a, p26) for which some supporting evidence has emerged (for example, O'Dwyer & Orrell, 1994).

Perhaps the most controversial of the four 'types of phenomena' in dementia which Kitwood (1989, pp4–7) held as being incompatible with the standard paradigm view is his notion of 'rementia'. Indeed, Kitwood acknowledged that when he first 'put forward the concept of "rementing", which many people have accepted now, it was tantamount to heresy' (Kitwood, 1997a, p4). This 'heresy' was first presented as the belief that 'Under certain circumstances sufferers from Alzheimer's Disease who had, apparently, gone far down the path of behavioural and cognitive impairment, can regain some of their lost faculties' (Kitwood, 1989, p5). Rementia typically consists of improved continence, along with 'moderate recoveries of memory, social skill, and ability to complete simple tasks, together with a general reduction of signs of anxiety' (ibid.).

The auspicious 'circumstances' equated, in essence, to good quality psychological care. Whilst it may be argued that an acceptance of the possibility of rementia is almost implied by an acceptance of the opinion that psychological and social factors play a real part in influencing the dementing process, the hostility it evoked in 1989 marks it out as being the most potent symbolic threat to the standard paradigm. Acceptance of the concept of rementia has profound implications for the relative ambitions of care and for the status of caregivers.

In addition to his criticisms of the empirical limitations of the standard paradigm, Kitwood was anxious to show that its representation of the nature of the relationship between mind and brain is quite untenable. We have already seen that the standard paradigm implies acceptance of an extreme form of reductionism, an absolute identification of 'mind' with 'brain' which holds that any change in one necessarily entails a corresponding change in the other — a change which would, at least in theory, be predictable. Kitwood dismissed such a position as being 'exceedingly difficult, if not impossible, to justify with logical rigour' (ibid., p3). And so research which restricts its horizons to studying neurological aspects alone, in the mistaken belief that the natural history of dementia is to be understood without reference to social or psychological factors, is inevitably incomplete: 'If the cause of the whole downward process of dementia is attributed to disease processes in the brain, we are no longer in the realm of science, but of neuropathic ideology' (Kitwood, 1997a, p67).

To move beyond that ideology, by formulating an understanding of the dementing process as part of the social and psychological context in which it occurs, is the challenge that Kitwood set for himself and for others of like mind. To those involved in dementia care it involves not only an attempt to reconceptualise dementia but also a re-evaluation of the task of caring, which moves, necessarily, 'beyond palliation' (ibid., p101) to an endeavour more akin to psychotherapy. Having accounted for the origins and shortcomings of the orthodox view of dementia, however, Kitwood's first task was to provide an alternative description, one which was drawn on a larger canvas, and took account of many more variables, than the standard paradigm was able to do.

A Reconceptualisation of Dementia

We referred earlier to the possibility that his stated objection to the standard paradigm could lead to Kitwood being misinterpreted as denying the role played by neuropathology in the process of dementia. In fact, he was very clear that there is a real pathology at work and that it does play a causal role in bringing about real neurological impairment. There were two key areas, however, that Kitwood did seek to challenge:

1 The perceived strength of the link between neuropathology and the symptoms of dementia.

2 The exclusion of other factors, particularly psychological and social factors, from our understanding of how dementia comes about and develops in any individual.

An appreciation of Kitwood's position is aided by a brief account of his ideas on the nature of language and on the nature of science. Kitwood referred to language as being like a type of net, or rather a series of nets, with which we endeavour to 'capture' as much reality as possible. Reality itself is infinitely complex, no language could ever hope to capture it completely, so we, as language-users, can only ever hope to capture an aspect of reality. A common mistake, however, is 'to take the descriptions and explanations given in language as if these were the reality itself' (Kitwood, 1997a, p17). This is something like the error at the heart of the standard paradigm, which asserts that the neuropathology it describes is the dementia, or the dementing process, which is in reality vastly more complex than the paradigm is able to allow for.

Kitwood referred to different language 'nets', or 'types of discourse', which operate according to their own rules and grammar and which have developed as being particularly suited to certain lines of enquiry. The natural sciences form one such 'type of discourse', with rules particularly suited to discovering some of the causal relationships that operate in nature. When it comes to assisting our understanding of human beings who inhabit worlds full of meaning and feeling, however, the natural sciences are restricted in their explanatory power and a fuller picture is provided by drawing on other disciplines. This limitation of the utility of the natural sciences led to the development of the 'human sciences', such as psychology and sociology, which operate within quite different rules from physics, or from biology. Whilst each has its own contribution to make in furthering our understanding of reality, Kitwood asserted that none can lay claim to having the sole authoritative voice with regard to dementia.

It is against this background that we can make sense of Kitwood's position on the role of neuropathology in dementia:

What is happening, and what has happened, when a person becomes demented in later life? In one gestalt configuration –

perhaps the prevailing one at present – the central figure is a process of degeneration, or some other physical impairment, in the grey matter of the brain; psychological and social factors fade into the background, at least for the purposes of research. Another gestalt, however, equally valid, can emerge; in this the figure becomes an existential crisis of a person, of an embodied, social and sentient being, and indeed a crisis of an interpersonal milieu; neuropathology, of whatever degree of severity, becomes part of a whole range of peripheral considerations.
(Kitwood, 1990b, p60)

Thus the objection to the standard paradigm view is not that it puts forward propositions that are false, but rather that it claims to paint a complete picture of dementia when, in reality, large parts are missing. This renders it unhelpful to our efforts in understanding any individual with dementia. Kitwood expressed what he believed to be a fuller, more helpful, outline of such a picture in the form of an equation:

$D = P + B + H + NI + SP$. This is simply to say that any individual's dementia (D) may be considered as the result of a complex interaction between five main components: personality (P), biography (B), physical health (H), neurological impairment (NI), and social psychology (SP).
(Kitwood, 1993a, p16)

We shall now look at each of these components in turn.

Personality
Kitwood's ideas on human personality development have roots in both the psychoanalytic and the person-centred traditions. When we look later at his use of the concept of 'personhood' we shall again encounter his belief that the maintenance, or dismantling, of personality in dementia is, essentially, a social process. Similarly, he argued, the formation of personality in infancy is ' … very clearly a social process, and not one of simple maturation' (Kitwood & Bredin, 1992a, p275).

Kitwood turned to David Winnicott, the psychoanalytically trained writer on child development, for an elucidation of the conditions determining the outcome of this social process of development. Winnicott summarised the requirements for an infant to develop a strong sense of self as a loving, caring environment and the encouragement of a sense of agency (conditions that re-emerge as part of Kitwood's requirements for the maintenance of self in dementia). A child growing up in a loving environment but who is repeatedly discouraged from showing signs of independence will fail to develop a sense of agency and, according to this view, will grow up to be very conforming and unadventurous.

Kitwood provided a neo-Rogerian account of the outcome of this developmental process in adult life, framed in terms of a distinction between an 'adapted self' and an 'experiential self'. Both selves:

> coexist 'within' any individual, and both … are socially formed. The experiential self is grounded in a kind of feeling–knowing or affectivity. It develops as experience is accepted, named and validated by others, and to the extent that a person can apprehend the self as an agent, one who creatively brings new things into being in the world. The adapted self has its basis in conformity to others' expectations, whether informally or in clearly structured roles.
> (Kitwood, 1990b, p61)

The concept of the experiential self has clear links with the Rogerian construct of the 'organismic self'. The individual in possession of a well-developed experiential self has a relatively high level of awareness of their experience and feelings. In Rogerian terms, they have a high level of congruence which, Kitwood asserted, makes them better equipped to cope with the losses that accompany dementia than one whose psychic defences remain high and inflexible.

Utilising another model, Kitwood gauged the modification of personality structure in terms of a continuum, illustrated as Figure 1. An individual's position on the continuum is determined by the extent and depth to which 'intersubjectivity' characterises their interpersonal relationships. 'Intersubjectivity' here has a meaning similar to Rogers' use of 'empathy', with its reference to the quality of psychological contact between individuals. The psyche that is surrounded by high and inflexible defences will remain in a 'frozen state' with relatively

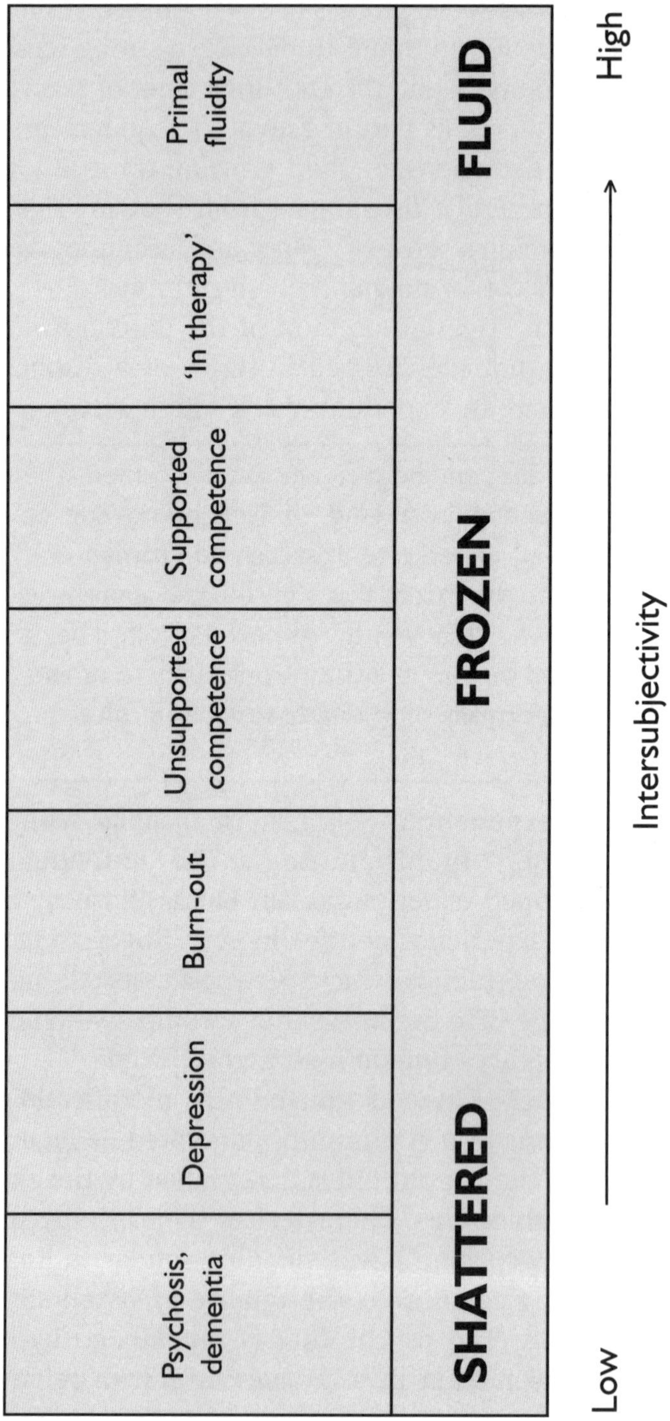

Low ——————→ High

Intersubjectivity

Source: Kitwood & Bredin (1992a, p277).

Figure 1 *Kitwood's Continuum Model of the Psyche*

low levels of intersubjectivity, whereas those who are able to lower defences, to 'let other people in', are said to be in a more fluid state. Those whose defences break down, and who are overwhelmed, find themselves unable to gain access to the quality of human contact they need and they occupy the 'shattered' end of the continuum.

Kitwood, clearly unimpressed by the efforts of orthodox psychology to capture the concept of personality, drew on ideas from a number of traditions in psychiatry and psychotherapy in his attempt to make sense of the personal characteristics people bring to the onset of a dementing illness. He understood personality as a set of resources and handicaps, acquired over a lifetime and constantly changing through experience. As a result he had little interest in addressing the question of whether personality 'changes' as a result of dementia — as it is in a constant state of flux anyway — although he viewed the tendency to include personality change as a symptom of dementia with considerable suspicion. Whilst changes may be witnessed in typical behaviours and in mood, Kitwood supported Bell and McGregor's (1995) assertion that these are more likely to be a consequence of an impoverished psychological environment than a direct result of neuropathology, with the exception of individuals who are known to have significant damage to the frontal lobes of the brain (Kitwood, 1997a, p31).

Biography
With the initial structure of personality set by the end of childhood, Kitwood believed its development in adult life is strongly influenced by the key, psychologically significant, events that contribute to each individual's biography. In the late 1980s, he conducted numerous lengthy interviews with family caregivers, gathering detailed accounts of the 'psychobiographies' of people with dementia (Kitwood, 1990b) which left him convinced that the course of a dementing illness is deeply interwoven with the psychosocial context in which it occurs. In particular, the history of the development of the 'adapted' and 'experiential' selves was seen as having a significant bearing on our ability to 'work through' the multiple losses which typically accompany old age and on how different individuals react to a decline in brain function. A host of factors — economic, social and political — were

cited as influencing the development of a psychobiography. In the case study of Rose (ibid.) Kitwood pointed to characteristics of the entire society, attributing a degree of responsibility for the underdevelopment of Rose's experiential self to the 'depredations brought about by the extraction of surplus value from wage labour' (ibid., p72) and to the 'social construction of gender' (ibid., p73). These, quasi-Marxist, aspects of his analysis point us towards a radical political element underlying Kitwood's position. When he referred to the psychological and social contexts in which a person's biography unfurls he was referring not only to the immediate interpersonal milieu but also to the wider politico-economic forces which help to shape that milieu.

Physical Health
Kitwood's area of expertise left him with little to say about physical health per se, but his holistic view of the mind–body relationship led him to speculate that both physical and psychological factors may be 'dementogenic'. The importance he attached to physical well-being is illustrated by his comment that 'Dementia … is always embedded in the general health picture of each individual … It is vital, then, that close attention be given to all aspects of the physical well-being of a person who has dementia' (Kitwood, 1997a, p34).

Neurological Impairment
We saw earlier that Kitwood's rejection of the explanation of dementia solely in terms of neuropathology did not amount to a denial of its role in bringing about neurological impairment. He accused the standard paradigm view of mistaking the relationship between neuropathology and clinical symptoms, between brain and mind, between neurology and psychology as being one of identification and of assuming that, in each case, the latter is ultimately reducible to the former. A better understanding of the relationship between brain and mind, Kitwood asserted, is provided by the notion of 'supervenience'. Mind, or a psychological state, can be conceived of as being a 'consequential characteristic' of a neurological state. In logical terms, supervenience refers to a property or quality that is dependent on some other quality or property, so that in this instance the psychological state would be

dependent on a particular brain state for its existence but should not be viewed as being identical with it. In this way he sought to avoid a dualist position, which treats 'mind' and 'matter' as each having a different kind of existence. Kitwood's monist position was maintained by his previously mentioned contention that psychology and neurology are two different types of discourse addressing what is, ultimately, the same reality. Thus any attempt to choose between a psychological and a neurological account of any mental process or event is misguided, as each is attempting to capture a different aspect (of the same process or event) according to the rules and conventions of its own subject. Each type of discourse has its own advantages and limitations and neither can claim to have an exclusive potential to capture the reality of its field of study. Kitwood employed symbols to articulate his position on the true relationship between mind and brain:

---

any psychological event (such as deciding to go for a walk) or state (such as feeling hungry) is also a brain event or state. It is not that the psychological event (ψ) is causing the brain activity (**b**) or vice versa; it is simply that some aspect of the true reality is being described in two different ways. Hence, in any individual, $\psi \equiv$ **b**. The 'equation' simply serves to emphasize the assumption that psychology and neurology are, in truth, inseparable.
(Kitwood, 1997a, p17)

The assumption that psychological/mental phenomena (ψ) are, in some fundamental way, caused by the state of the brain (**b**) is a deeply entrenched habit of much of western psychiatric thought. Kitwood asks us to consider an example in which neurological impairment is not thought to be involved: suppose a person is in an agitated distressed state, with a psychological state $\psi 1$ and a brain state **b1**.This person may go to a doctor and be prescribed a sedative which takes him to psychological state $\psi 2$ and brain state **b2**. He may, on the other hand, spend an hour with a skilled counsellor and, for the purposes of this example, end up with exactly the same psychological state $\psi 2$ and brain state **b2**. This simple, relatively uncontroversial, example illustrates how the change from state $\psi 1 \equiv$ **b1** to state $\psi 2 \equiv$ **b2** can occur either through medication, which would usually be having a causal effect on the brain state (**b**), or through counselling, which would usually be thought of as having an impact on the psychological state (ψ). In either instance, the brain state and the psychological state change at the same time because, in reality, they are the same thing. It is because of this idea of the ultimate unity of mind and brain that Kitwood described his position as 'monist', as opposed to the standard paradigm's 'dualist' position which implies a duality of mind and brain, with one phenomenon (brain) 'causing' changes in the other (mind).

The implications of this monist view for Kitwood's conceptualisation of the relationship between neuropathology and dementia now become clearer. He again expressed his position by the use of symbols (ibid., p18), emphasising the emerging view from neuroscience that the structure of the brain continues to develop throughout life and that this development (Bd) must also be taken into account in dementia, alongside brain pathology (Bp):

$$\frac{\psi \equiv \mathbf{b}}{(Bd, Bp)}$$

(Any psychological event or state is also a brain event or state, 'carried' by a brain whose structure has been determined by both developmental and pathological factors.)

In relation to the causes of neurological impairment, we have already witnessed Kitwood's insistence that we should not move beyond the evidence regarding the relationship of brain structure and neurological impairment, or brain function. After tentatively advancing the suggestion that 'Malignant Social Psychology', discussed below, may play a causal role in bringing about neurological impairment (Kitwood, 1990a, p18) Kitwood was partially vindicated by research linking the onset of dementia with stress. Subsequently, it became central to his position that psychological aspects of the environment may well be as 'dementogenic' as physical factors, including any 'factor X' which may (or may not) emerge as the causal agent behind the neuropathology of Alzheimer's Disease.

So how might psychological events, such as episodes of stress produced by a malignant social psychology, actually cause structural changes to the brain? To Kitwood such a question is grounded in dualist thinking, to be met by his urging us to remember that each psychological event, such as a session of counselling or a period of stress, is also an event in the brain. We can then postulate that, over time, such events might accumulate to produce organic, structural changes, such as those associated with dementia. It may be in the same kind of way that the flow of a river will, over time, alter the structure of the terrain through which it passes. Indeed, the distinction between brain function and brain structure should not be exaggerated: 'Function might be regarded as 'fast process of short duration', and structure as 'slow process of long duration'' (Kitwood, 1989, p8).

Social Psychology
Most of us will arrive at the onset of dementia with a personality that is already formed and a biography that has been largely developed. Despite recent pharmacological advances, we continue to have little influence over the pathological contribution to neurological impairment and Kitwood offered nothing new in respect of physical health. It is not surprising, therefore, that in his role as a theorist of dementia care he reserved most attention for social psychology, as it is on this final 'component' of dementia that the quality of care can have the most significant impact, for better or for worse. The following section looks in more detail at the powerful effect that, Kitwood believed, social psychology has on the person with dementia.

The Social Psychology of Dementia
Kitwood's eloquent exposition of the insight that social psychology can bring to the world of dementia care accounts for much of the impact and appeal of his work. Just as Goffman managed to articulate the reality of life in the asylums — a reality of which many had a diffuse, uneasy, awareness — so Kitwood held up a mirror to the situation surrounding people with dementia. That this induced a collective sense of shame may be indicative of the potential for future improvement. It is also testament to Kitwood's ability to ensure that our reflection, as

99

carers, is included alongside that of the person with dementia, and we are not flattered by many of the things it reveals.

Social psychology has been described as a discipline which is 'continually inter-relating three levels of analysis, the individual, the interpersonal and the social structural (which should be taken to include political and economic structures)' (Fraser, 1987, p721). With this in mind, we ought not to be surprised by Kitwood's insistence that any account of dementia that gives genuine consideration to those psychological and social factors that shape it will come not 'from the standpoint of a narrow individualism, but from a genuinely social perspective' (Kitwood, 1990b, p61).

For Kitwood, society is as culpable for the lack of 'intersubjective insight' in our interpersonal relationships as it is for the burdens and pressure it places on caregivers by its failure to provide sufficient resources for care. On a social–structural level, dominant belief systems affect the immediate social milieu of the person with dementia. They promote the widely held belief that people with dementia cease, on some level, to be a person at all (Kitwood, 1990a, pp184–185), as dementia leaves behind a 'shell' of a person while robbing the sufferer of those essential features that make us human. Such attitudes collude with the standard paradigm, giving carers permission to disengage emotionally from the person with dementia, justifying the belief that 'How I relate to this person matters little as their deterioration is inevitable and they are no longer really present anyway.'

Emphasising the influence which society has in shaping the experience of the individual with dementia may appear to lead towards the conclusion that significant improvement is possible only through a transformation of society as a whole. Kitwood appeared, however, to see the relationship between society and individual as being less deterministic than that conclusion would imply, and his focus was more on the immediate interpersonal environment of the person with dementia. The Bradford Dementia Group has devoted considerable amounts of time and effort attempting to identify the features of that environment that may be available for measurement and for modification — a concentration of effort that is consistent with the degree of influence on 'personhood' that Kitwood attributed to the psychosocial environment.

Personhood

Reference has already been made to Kitwood's belief that a person's subjective appreciation of themselves as a single being, with a continuous thread of subjective experience, is an outcome of early social relationships: 'Putting it another way, relationship comes first, and with it intersubjectivity; the subjectivity of the individual is like a distillate that is collected later' (Kitwood & Bredin, 1992a, p275). Our sense of self, or selfhood, is more or less robust, depending on the quality of those early relationships, especially those involving our primary caregivers. Where it is in a reasonable condition it assures us that we are, on a fundamental level, a continuation of the same person that we were yesterday and that tomorrow, notwithstanding the modifications that each of us undergoes each day, we shall be the same person again. This experience of the continuity of self can be contrasted to the individual who is experiencing a fragmentation of their psyche, as in a psychosis, or to one who is in a state of extreme alienation from their experience. In such cases the sense of perspective and continuity regarding the relationship of past, present and future experiences has become extremely disjointed, or may even be absent.

There is a strong temptation to describe a reasonably integrated adult psyche as largely self-maintaining, developing largely according to an internal dynamic, with little influence attributed to the interpersonal environment. The most common modes of behaviour in our society reinforce this view. Predictable daily behaviour patterns and the ability to carry through long-term projects, either in work or when engaging in leisure, sustain an image of continuity that collapses only in the face of 'personal' crises. This is, Kitwood believed, a temptation to be resisted. For him the self that is created in relationship is also maintained in relationship, albeit in adulthood those relationships are usually more diverse and complex than that between primary caregiver and infant. In recognition of this social requirement for the maintenance of selfhood, Kitwood used the term 'personhood', after the Swiss psychologist, Paul Tournier:

> Personhood ... requires a living relationship with at least one other, where there is a felt bond, or tie. Without this as a minimum

> the human psyche disintegrates, except in the most exceptional
> cases. It is also necessary for an individual to have some place of
> significance within a human grouping, bound together on the basis
> of family, friendship, occupation, religion, neighbourhood or
> whatever. It is as if the group comes to exist in the individual, as
> well as the individual within the group.
> (Kitwood, 1997b, p11)

The concept of personhood calls into question the distinction between the 'internal' and 'external' worlds of the individual, a distinction that was, for Kitwood, symptomatic of the individualistic ideology that pervades western societies. Thus 'subjectivity' cannot be maintained without 'intersubjectivity' to nourish it. Our profoundly social nature is such that alienation from our fellow humans leads invariably, albeit at variable pace, to alienation from our own selves. This mutual dependency may be disguised for considerable amounts of time by the adult psyche that is built on firm foundations, carrying sufficient resources, but it is openly revealed by the need for intersubjectivity displayed by the infant building up their own subjectivity and by the older person with failing mental powers who is struggling to maintain theirs.

If personhood is to be maintained, an individual needs not only relationships but also to be accorded status. In ethics, and in law, that status is of a fellow human being entitled to the same degree of respect and consideration as any other. In terms of social status, it requires an acknowledgement of one's subjectivity and uniqueness as an individual (Kitwood, 1997b).

The degree of respect afforded to one's subjectivity is, of course, extremely variable. It can be affirmed or denied according to the social milieu in which the individual is situated. In everyday language, its affirmation can be summed up as those experiences in which someone feels they have been affirmed, or 'treated like a real person', with their feelings acknowledged and their point of view valued. The denial of personhood, on the other hand, is experienced through contact with people who do not fully acknowledge your presence, when people act as if you are not there or treat you as if you are not worthy of their full attention and consideration. In everyday interpersonal interaction any individual can expect to have their personhood affirmed or denied, in varying degrees, many times in the course of a normal day, during which most of us will, equally, affirm or deny the personhood of others. Events at this interpersonal, or 'microsocial', level are clearly influenced by the predominant social relations that characterise the social structural level. Thus any enterprise that is organised as a hierarchy will, we can say with some confidence, have an inbuilt tendency to encourage greater respect for the personhood of those who occupy positions nearer its apex than it does for those at its base. Similarly, most interactions which involve the purchase of goods or, more especially, of a service will tend to involve greater accord being given to the subjectivity of the purchaser than it is to that of the provider. We know what response to expect if we question a restaurant owner, for example, if they are more concerned about the way the staff or the customers feel at the end of an evening, and we know the reason they will give. The customers must want to come back again, to ensure profits are maintained. The staff are being paid, and their feelings matter only in so far as they affect their ability to behave in a way that keeps the customer happy.

Kitwood described the work of the Jewish religious philosopher Martin Buber as 'Perhaps the most profound account of personhood in this century' (Kitwood, 1997b, p4). Buber, one of the leading Jewish intellectuals in Germany during the inter-war years, published a short book entitled *I and Thou* in 1922. It contains:

---

his philosophy of dialogue, a religious existentialism centered on the distinction between direct, mutual relations (called by him the 'I–Thou' relationship, or dialogue), in which each person confirms the other as of unique value, and indirect, utilitarian relations (designated the 'I–It' relationship, or monologue), in which each person knows and uses others but does not really see or value them for themselves.
(Friedman, 1994)

In Kitwood's eyes, this distinction captures the essence of the manner in which the nature of our relationships can serve either to enhance or diminish our personhood. I–Thou encounters will always replenish personhood and subjectivity. They involve lowering our defences and allowing our true feelings to show, secure in the knowledge that they will be affirmed and respected. They are the deepest relationships that humans are capable of yet they are, tragically, something of a rarity in a society whose structures positively discriminate in favour of I–It relationships. Kitwood picked out the assumptions underlying the academic discipline of western psychology — with its aspiration for the kind of objective rigour that characterises the natural sciences — as having 'no place for the I-Thou mode of relating' (Kitwood, 1997b, p6); 'The great exception of course, is psychotherapy ... In therapeutic work, despite many failures and abuses, there is a serious commitment to meeting' (Kitwood, 1997b, p7).

In dementia, as in psychosis, it is the experience of a 'continuing line of selfhood' that Kitwood believed to be in danger of fragmentation. With dementia, however, the prevalence of the 'standard paradigm' has led many of us to make the invalid inference that loss of selfhood, the disintegration of the personality, is an inevitable result of neuropathological processes. We have seen how, for Kitwood, intersubjectivity — that personal affirmation provided by good quality psychological contact — nourishes personhood and this makes it all the more necessary when personhood comes under threat from neuropathology. Kitwood was therefore witness to a genuine tragedy when he saw the quality of the interpersonal milieu surrounding the person with dementia changing in exactly the opposite way to that which was required. Instead of the social psychology becoming rich in empathy, acceptance and support, he saw the formation of a phenomenon which he christened the 'Malignant Social Psychology' (MSP) — a typical, distinctive and unhelpful set of reactions amongst those who surround the person with dementia which have the effect of combining with neurological impairment to set up a vicious cycle of decline. MSP is inimical to the replenishment of personhood. Whilst those who are cognitively intact may instinctively recognise a social psychology which is malignant, take steps to avoid it, and/or organise the replenishment of their personhood elsewhere, those with dementia are generally captive to their social situation. They are able only to withdraw or to protest at the attenuation of their personhood with whatever resources are available. In either event, if caregivers fail to attend to their subjectivity the results, Kitwood suggested, will be inevitable: 'in 'unattended dementia' there is a dismantling of personality, a loss of self' (Kitwood, 1990c, p48).

Kitwood was fortunate in having evidence close at hand which suggested that an environment that is rich in personhood-enhancing features could actively prevent this 'loss of self'. Janet Bell and Iain McGregor had already established Spring Mount Residential Home in Bradford as a radical departure from orthodox care facilities for people with dementia. Their work, which will be described more fully later, was founded on a determination to eradicate the use of tranquillising medication, combined with the creation of a supportive and enabling social environment. They were witness to results that challenged the notion that this 'loss of self' was inevitably concomitant with dementia. Bell and McGregor were able to assure Kitwood that 'every single person in our care has proved to be a unique individual. Despite the commonly held belief that dementia destroys personality, they have retained the basic core characteristics that made them the person they always were' (Bell & McGregor, 1995, p12).

Such anecdotal reports serve as counter-evidence to the claim that dementia is a disease which involves an inevitable progression to a 'severe' stage in which individuals lose all contact with the social environment and become unresponsive. They suggest the possibility that it was that very environment that rendered them thus, even in the event of discovering comparatively greater neurological damage which might, in fact, be explained as effect rather than cause. While this possibility remains alive (and it is difficult to see how it could possibly be removed) the starting point for maintaining personhood is to be found in the social psychology of the immediate, interpersonal, milieu. This explains Kitwood's devoting so much attention to categorising those characteristics of the social psychology that surrounds dementia sufferers, to developing methods to measure it and to suggesting strategies to improve it.

The Malignant Social Psychology
It will be noticed that there has been a shift in the use of the phrase 'social psychology'. We began by referring to it as an academic

discipline, an area of study, and have moved to discussing it as if it were some kind of entity. Kitwood tended to focus on the latter usage, for him it refers to a crucial aspect of our environment: 'human beings are far more deeply affected by the social psychology that surrounds them than is commonly recognised ... When a person has been subjected to a predominantly malignant social psychology for several years, the effects may indeed be devastating' (Kitwood, 1990a, p181).

What kind of 'thing' is this social psychology which 'surrounds' us? It is best understood as shorthand for 'social–psychological milieu' (ibid., p178). The aspects of the milieu which can be said to define the social psychology are those that affect us directly, through our experiencing them, and those that affect our status, the results of which we experience indirectly. The degree to which individuals are consciously aware of that experience will vary. Thus when Kitwood referred to the 'malignant social psychology', he was pointing to a set of characteristic aspects of interpersonal interactions and relationships which are perceived as damaging to the personhood of the person with dementia. In another of Kitwood's models for understanding dementia, MSP is held to be one of the factors which combines in a 'dialectical relationship' with neurological impairment to produce senile dementia, a proposition which Kitwood (ibid., p180) included in his theory of dementia as the first of three equations:

$$SD = NI + MSP$$

Senile Dementia is compounded from the effects of Neurological Impairment and of Malignant Social Psychology.

The initial description of the malignancy surrounding dementia sufferers (Kitwood, 1990a) consisted of 10 characteristic behaviours displayed by carers and professionals. To these a further seven were added later (Kitwood, 1997a). They are summarised in Table 3.

Caregivers tend to recognise the examples provided by Kitwood as illustrations of each aspect of MSP (Kitwood, 1990a, pp181–184) as commonplace features of the lives of people with dementia. He was keen to stress that, although the malignancy consists of the behaviour of those surrounding the person with dementia, it is seldom created as

Table 3 *Kitwood's Malignant Social Psychology*

Aspect	Description
Accusation	The person is blamed for action, or failure to act, which results from their loss of skills or inability to understand the situation.
Banishment	The person is either sent away or excluded — either physically, psychologically, or both — thus depriving them of sustaining human contact.
Disempowerment	The person is not allowed to utilise their remaining abilities. They do not receive assistance to complete actions they have initiated.
Disparagement	The person is given messages that they are incompetent, a failure and so on. This damages their self-esteem.
Disruption	The person experiences a sudden disturbance to their frame of reference while in the middle of an action or reflection.
Ignoring	Carrying on conversation or actions as if the person were not present.
Imposition	Overriding the desires of, or denying choice to, a person.
Infantilisation	Treating a person very patronisingly, as if they were a young child.
Intimidation	A person is made fearful by threats, physical power or by being placed in situations in which they are unable to make sense of their surroundings.
Invalidation	The person's subjectivity, especially their feelings, is either denied, not acknowledged or dismissed as insignificant.
Labelling	The diagnostic category becomes the foundation for attempts to understand, and attempts to communicate with, a person.
Mockery	A person's disabilities are used as a source of humour.

Objectification	A person's status as a sentient human being is disregarded. They are treated as if they are not really present.
Outpacing	A person is excluded by those around them acting and speaking at a pace which leaves them bewildered.
Stigmatisation	The person is treated as an outcast.
Treachery	Trickery and deception are used in order to manipulate a person into behaving in a way that is desired by others.
Withholding	A person's physical and psychological needs are disregarded.

Source: Adapted from Kitwood (1990a, pp181–184; 1997a, pp46–47).

a result of malicious intent. Rather, it is part of the cultural inheritance of dementia care, consisting largely of behaviours that occur 'without thinking' or with some justification, such as the 'ends justify the means'. A common thread linking all the behaviours of the MSP is the disregard they show towards the subjectivity of the person with dementia. Things are not done deliberately in order to hurt or to demoralise, but our sensitivity as to what may hurt or demoralise becomes greatly diminished. Placed in a social context in which the degree of sensitivity shown towards the experience of others is, at best, somewhat variable, any decline in intersubjectivity involving people with dementia constitutes a serious threat to their already fragile personhood.

We saw earlier how each psychological event, in this case characterised by MSP, also involves an accompanying neurological event. Thus the MSP and the neuropathology 'meet' at the neurological level, with neurological consequences. These, in turn, create social–psychological consequences, as the resultant behavioural changes of the dementia sufferer induce further malignant responses from those that surround them. Kitwood described this relationship between the psychological effects of the MSP and the consequences of neuropathology as a 'dialectic'. By this he meant that the process of dementia involves two tendencies — in this case neurological impairment and MSP — influencing a situation so as to create a new situation which is, in turn, affected by the same two tendencies so that a third situation is developed. A typical example of a dialectical 'vicious circle' at work in dementia is summarised by Kitwood as a diagram, reproduced below as Figure 2, in which 'NI' refers to 'Neurological Impairment'.

The attraction to Kitwood's work amongst those involved in caring for people with dementia is enhanced by his descriptions of many aspects of their daily lives. He also appeals to a strongly felt sense that our mental lives are not determined by internal factors alone, without reference to either our social environment or the significant events in our lives. This is where the standard paradigm, as Kitwood portrayed it, breaks down. The relative strength of Kitwood's exposition lies in its breadth and also in the clear implications that it has for care. Whereas the standard paradigm condemns carers to the position of a passive witness, the dialectical model makes them key players, able to influence the course of the dementia — either for better or for worse.

Before we go on to look at some of the implications for care, however, it is worth briefly noting one observation on the collective 'social structural' position of people with dementia. There are noticeable parallels between Kitwood's dialectical model of dementia and the notions of the disabling environment — characterised by the disabling effects of other people's attitudes — which has been an intellectual cornerstone of the struggle of people within the disabilities movement in recent decades. Janet Bell and Iain McGregor have incorporated this identification of dementia as a (potentially multiple) disability as a fundamental tenet of their philosophy at Spring Mount, a conceptual move that encourages us to push the dementia to one side and allows the person to occupy the forefront of our appreciation.

Well-Being in Dementia

To accept Kitwood's entreaty to revise our notion of dementia is to acknowledge the need to reappraise our ideas of well-being, if they are to complement the broader view of dementia that we have come to hold. 'Relative well-being' (Kitwood & Bredin, 1992a) in dementia is

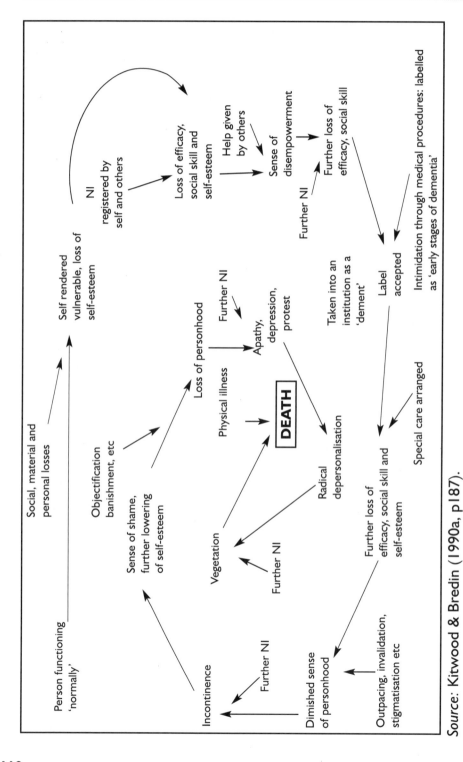

Source: Kitwood & Bredin (1990a, p187).

Figure 2 *Kitwood's Model of the Dementing Process*

concerned with personhood maintained, rather than with minimising impairment. It is related to emotional experience, personality, self-esteem, creativity and other characteristics assumed to have the potential to remain relatively unscathed by the disease process. Kitwood and Bredin's list of 'twelve indicators of well-being' (summarised in Table 4), is based on this assumption, that deterioration in each indicator is more likely to be a function of MSP than it is to be part of any globalised deterioration resulting from neuropathology alone.

Kitwood equated well-being with the maintenance of personhood, arguing that the indicators contained in Table 4 are expressions of 'four apprehensions or global sentient states , , a sense of personal worth ... a sense of agency ... social confidence ... [and] hope' (ibid., pp282–283). These four 'apprehensions' might accompany a well-maintained personhood in anyone, regardless of their cognitive status. Indeed, any individual enjoying all four consistently would clearly be in

Table 4 *Kitwood & Bredin's Twelve Indicators of Well-being in Dementia*
The assertion of desire or will
The ability to experience and express a range of emotions
Initiation of social contact
Affectional warmth
Social sensitivity
Self-respect
Acceptance of other dementia sufferers
Humour
Creativity and self-expression
Showing evident pleasure
Helpfulness
Relaxation
Source: Adapted from Kitwood & Bredin (1992a, pp281–282).

the best of psychological health. Kitwood made no apology for judging the well-being of people with dementia in such general terms, freely acknowledging that 'The indicators … are part of the common ground between those who are and who are not dementing' (ibid., p282).

Although Kitwood was reluctant to include cognitive factors in his identification of well-being, he was willing to suggest that a good care environment may well have beneficial effects in this regard: 'perhaps slowing down the pathological processes and enhancing growth in the neurones that remain' (Kitwood, 1997a, p69). As before, this should not be misinterpreted as Kitwood stating that psychological causes are bringing about neurological effects, but rather as his considering possible neurological concomitants of a process that is being described in its psychological aspect.

Kitwood proposed that the satisfaction of five psychological 'needs' is required for a person with dementia to attain a state of well-being. These needs — attachment, psychological comfort, a sense of identity, occupation and inclusion in groups (ibid., pp81–84) — are said to be common to all humans, but are heightened by the experience of dementia. The disabilities associated with dementia often make them more difficult to attain and the goal of Kitwood's notion of 'person-centred' dementia care can be seen as an attempt to compensate for this deficit.

Person-Centred Dementia Care

As we might expect in the light of his understanding of dementia, Kitwood believed we can learn much from the various psychotherapeutic traditions to assist our attempt to discern the nature of good quality dementia care. Whilst his earlier articles on dementia drew some rather generalised conclusions about the characteristics of care, from 1992 he was much concerned with dementia care as it is delivered in the real world. As a result, many people found that their ideas on the desirable characteristics of caregivers were radically altered.

The Lessons from Psychotherapy

There are strong echoes of Rogers in Kitwood's insistence that there can be no interpersonal 'techniques' in dementia care which will substitute for therapeutic relationships of quality and depth, and I have noted in

Chapter 1 the indifference to cognitive functioning contained in Rogers' explanation of the therapeutic relationship. Although accounts of the therapeutic process are notoriously contentious, many would share the view that the process of successful psychotherapy consists of two individuals forming a relationship which allows one of them (the client) to restructure, or modify, their mental world. The therapist is often seen as fulfilling sufficient of the client's emotional needs (for acceptance and validation) to allow them to incorporate a greater part of their (internal and external) experience into consciousness. The key aspects of the process, then, are the relationships between therapist and client and between the client and their own experience. Kitwood was able to claim some support from the analytic as well as the person-centred tradition for his claim that we should attach 'relatively little weight to cognition, and ... [regard] ... the whole process as fundamentally relational (Symington, 1988:25–38)' (Kitwood, 1997a, p98).

The fact of cognitive impairment will, however, have implications for the way in which any therapeutic relationship is achieved and maintained. Like Goudie and Stokes, Kitwood was well aware that the traditional weekly one-hour session would not suffice, and that we should have to think in terms of a psychotherapeutic environment, as opposed to a one-to-one relationship (notwithstanding that there would be room for individual therapeutic relationships within the care milieu). In therapeutic terms, Kitwood summarised the difference from therapy with those without cognitive impairment:

The sufferer from dementia has a memory problem, and generally it is much harder for him or her to retain the image of those who are helping with containment. As with the very young child, there is a much greater need for the container to be visibly, tangibly, reliably present, and for longer periods of time. It is as if the rapid-acting, snapshot-taking part of the mental apparatus has failed; but the slow acting part – operating more like the silver film in the earliest experiments in photography, which acquired an image slowly and indistinctly – still functions. Although clear-cut cognitive memory is not present, an emotional memory survives.
(Kitwood, 1990c, p50)

Whereas Resolution Therapy drew attention to the potential for adapting some of the skills employed in Person-Centred Therapy, Kitwood was more concerned with a person-centred emphasis on the therapeutic relationship. His acknowledgement that such relationships are a kind of love (Kitwood, 1997a, p81) would find support amongst some of the inheritors of the person-centred tradition (for example, Brazier, 1993). We can also interpret his call to reframe our relationships with people with dementia, by acknowledging the contribution that we (the cognitively intact) bring to the problem, as a plea for greater congruence.

Reference has already been made to the central place that empathy occupied in Kitwood's theory of dementia care, although he tended to prefer to use terms such as 'intersubjectivity' and 'intersubjective insight' which have their origins in social psychology. He was keen to erode the pessimism that had attached itself to the possibility of achieving insight into the experience of dementia, whilst recognising that such insight always had its limitations. He described seven 'access routes' (Kitwood, 1997a, pp73–79), proposing that we can enhance our appreciation of the experience of dementia by reading accounts by people who have dementia; by listening to their attempts to describe their experience; by being alert to the possibility that everyday speech contains metaphors of their experience; by being alert to the messages contained in the behaviour of people with dementia; by hearing the recollections of those who have recovered from reversible dementia-like illnesses, such as meningitis or depression; through the use of our own 'poetic imagination' and, finally, through role-play. While each of these has its limitations, taken together Kitwood believed they are the best attempt we can make to appreciate the subjective world of the person with dementia.

It would be misleading to create the impression that the lessons Kitwood drew from psychotherapy are from the person-centred tradition alone, notwithstanding the significant contribution that it makes. Such an impression could be reinforced by the fact that Kitwood chose to describe his approach to care as 'person-centred' and it is worth noting, therefore, that in using this term he did not intend to imply either an approach that is exclusively Rogerian, or one derived exclusively from Rogerian principles. His account of the development of personhood, for example, was informed by the views of the psychoanalytically orientated David Winnicott, and his approaches to dementia, to care and to caring organisations were all founded on an understanding of dynamics, utilising concepts such as 'psychic defences' that belong very much to the various psychodynamic traditions. Kitwood made no apologies for drawing upon the insights of a wide range of thinkers in order to make sense of his experiences of working with dementia. Doing so was consistent with his view of the relationship between language and reality, the view that all the various traditions have evolved different vocabularies to describe what is, ultimately, the same thing, and that none of them can claim an exclusive insight into the 'truth' of the human condition.

From Theory to Practice
Throughout the first half of the 1990s, Kitwood's agenda was set by his identification of the 'Malignant Social Psychology' as a contributory factor in dementia. Having 'discovered' a profoundly negative influence on the quality of care, it is understandable that the bulk of his work was then committed to the task of reducing, even eliminating, that influence. As a consequence, the emphasis was very much on the negative effects of poor quality care, with less attention paid to the specifics of good care. This emphasis was reflected in the earlier versions of Dementia Care Mapping (discussed later in this chapter) and in the guide for carers produced with Kathleen Bredin (Kitwood & Bredin, 1992b) which, although a useful summary of current best practice, had little that was particularly innovative to suggest about the way in which care is delivered. The Bradford Group had reached a stage in which they had considerable expertise in advising caregivers what to avoid, and were clearly needing to develop their own vision of what carers should actually be doing. Kitwood was to discover that 'Even where malignant social psychology has been almost totally eliminated it is rare to find that the space has been filled by a social psychology that is thoroughly empowering and sustaining' (Kitwood, 1997a, p87).

Having developed the tools that could enable carers to stop doing harm to people with dementia, the logical next contribution was towards equipping them with the skills, knowledge and working environment that would allow them to make positive therapeutic gains. Kitwood moved towards this end with his development of a description of 'positive person work' (ibid., pp89–93) which serves as the 'helpful' counterpart of the Malignant Social Psychology. He also, in line with the principles of social psychology, devoted increasing attention to the organisational and developmental aspects of the care environment (see, for example, ibid., pp103–107) which will not be looked at in any detail here. Suffice it to say that he drew attention to the need for organisations concerned with care to 'nourish the subjectivity' of care staff at a time when both the public and independent sectors were dominated by a managerial culture that barely acknowledged the possibility of such a need being appropriate to their agenda. We can discern in Kitwood's writings on the organisation of care another link with Rogers, who also accepted the view that therapists/carers cannot be reasonably expected to meet the needs of a client/person with dementia if their own needs are being disregarded. Kitwood also addressed the issue of 'cultural transformation' (for example, Kitwood, 1995; 1997a, pp133–144), proposing steps that individuals and organisations can take in order to shift from the 'old culture of dementia care' (which remains steeped in the values implicit in the standard paradigm) to a new culture which has grown since the mid-1980s in spite of the sociostructural obstacles that were laid in its path.

Rogers refused to limit the application of his approach to understanding the individual in therapy and sought to apply his ideas to a wider, even international, context, especially in his later years. Kitwood remained concerned with dementia care but acknowledged that the principles which underlie the relationship between carer and cared-for also apply to the relationship between organisation and carer. This point is crucial to our avoiding the erroneous conclusion that Kitwood's work simply involved a shift in the designation of the 'problem' from the person with dementia to the caregiver. That conclusion was certainly drawn by some who read his earlier work, especially that on the MSP, and were led to seek a 'managerialist' solution, consisting solely of 'educating' carers and 'selecting' the right staff. While Kitwood agreed that these are parts of the solution, his later work was clear that the 'requirements of a caregiver' cannot be viewed in isolation from 'the caring organization' (Kitwood, 1997a, pp103–132).

At the microsocial, face-to-face, level at which care is delivered, the quality of the relationship with the caregiver is deemed to have the most potential for a beneficial effect on personhood. Clearly the attitude of the caregiver will be a paramount concern, but there are also, Kitwood asserted, important skills to be acquired if carers are to engage successfully in 'positive person work'. These are primarily interpersonal skills which are not to be confused with the interpersonal 'techniques' associated with some other approaches. A basic skill in dementia care is an ability to communicate, to retain contact, in the face of advancing expressive and receptive dysphasia. One of Kitwood's first steps upon shifting his attention from a general theory of dementia to the specifics of dementia care was to apply a triadic model of communication to our understanding of communication and dementia (Kitwood, 1993b). Rejecting the conventional 'Morse code model' (which involves a sender encoding a message which is decoded by a receiver) as inadequate to capture the subtleties of human communication, he borrowed a model from symbolic interactionism, based on the reflexive triad, outlined in Table 5. Where such triads involve a person whose cognitions are damaged, a suitable therapeutic response from a caregiver is outlined in Table 6. Whilst the triadic model helps to elucidate the form of therapeutic interventions in dementia, their content is categorised by the list of positive interactions which enhance personhood, and these are summarised in Table 7. This list is in contrast to the 17 behaviours of the Malignant Social Psychology which attenuate personhood.

Kitwood did not claim that the list in Table 7 is exhaustive and, while his own concern was primarily with improving the social psychology surrounding people with dementia, he did not seek to imply that this was the only way in which the quality of life for people with dementia can be enriched. Indeed, he cited a number of other factors which have contributed to the 'almost revolutionary' improvements in care since the mid-1980s: 'We have better methods of assessment, positive care planning, a rich and varied range of activities, a commitment to the needs of people rather than of

Table 5 *The Reflexive Triad*

Person X	(a) with their own given temperament, constitution, etc,
	(b) carrying their unique legacy from past experience,
	(c) in a particular sentient state (regarding mood, emotion, feeling etc),
	(d) defines the situation in a certain way and
	(e) having various assumptions (about the expectations of others and their states),
	(f) with certain desires, intentions, expectations, etc,
	makes an action.
Person Y	(a) with their own given temperament, constitution, etc,
	(b) carrying their unique legacy from past experience,
	(c) in a particular sentient state (regarding mood, emotion, feeling etc),
	(d) defines the situation in a certain way and
	(e) having various assumptions (about the expectations of others and their states),
	interprets Person X's action and
	(f) with certain desires, intentions, expectations, etc
	responds.
Person X	Interprets Person Y's response and
	reflects,
	checking in various ways whether the act she or he is trying to bring off with Person Y is likely to be successful.

Source: Adapted from Kitwood (1993b, p56).

institutional regimes, purpose-built physical environments, and many other huge improvements' (Kitwood, 1997a, p86).

Although too many care environments remain untouched by these advances, there has been sufficient progress to justify Kitwood's heralding the arrival of a 'new culture of dementia care' (for example, Kitwood, 1995). His influence on the form that this new culture has taken is such that it is difficult to imagine any service aspiring to be part

Table 6 *Therapeutic Responses from Caregivers*

Person X, who has dementia

makes a gesture: an utterance of some kind, or a bodily movement.

The caregiver

recognises Person X's gesture and honours it with a response;

has some empathic understanding of Person X's inwardly 'shattered' state;

has some sense of what Person X might be experiencing;

fills out a definition of the situation in collaboration with Person X;

appreciates and responds to the desire or need that Person X may be expressing, helping to convert it into an intention;

uses interaction to sustain Person X's action, preventing it falling into the void as a result of Person X's memory deficit;

responds sensitively to signs that Person X's proto-definition of the situation might be changing, and moves with that change;

'holds' Person X through whatever emotional experience the interaction may entail, so that it becomes a completed act in the social world.

Source: Adapted from Kitwood (1993b, p58).

of it without expressing an ambition to meet emotional needs and to address the experience of those in its care. In this context, it is worth noting that many of those who advocate the adoption of a person-centred approach to dementia care do so with a tacit acknowledgement of the influence of Kitwood, rather than that of Rogers.

Dementia Care Mapping

The influence of the British renaissance in dementia care on services remains uneven, and ideas of what constitutes an 'advance' in dementia care remain far from shared. It was partly as a response to this situation that Kitwood progressed from his identification of social psychology as the 'crucial variable' in dementia care to developing a method which might go some way towards evaluating the quality of

Table 7 *Kitwood's 'Positive Person Work'*

Aspect	Description
Recognition	In which the person with dementia is acknowledged as a person, affirmed in his or her own uniqueness.
Negotiation	In which people with dementia are consulted about their preferences, desires and needs.
Collaboration	In which the person with dementia's own initiative and abilities are involved.
Play	Involving spontaneity and self-expression that has value in itself.
Timalation	Which is primarily sensuous or sensual, without the involvement of the intellect.
Celebration	In which the division between caregiver and cared-for comes nearest to vanishing completely.
Relaxation	Which can be done in isolation but which many people with dementia prefer to do with others near.
Validation	In which the reality and power of the person with dementia's experiences are acknowledged.
Holding	Providing a safe psychological 'space' in which hidden trauma and conflict can be brought out.
Facilitation	Enabling interaction to begin, amplifying it and helping the person with dementia fill it out with meaning.

Source: Adapted from Kitwood (1997a, pp90–91).

that social psychology. As the administrator of the Bradford Dementia Group, Linda Fox, has expressed it: 'If it is really the case that a new culture in dementia care is emerging, we need means to identify how far this has come about. Dementia Care Mapping (known as DCM) is one such method' (Fox, 1995, p70).

Dementia Care Mapping aims to identify, in some detail, any progress that services make in moving away from the old culture of dementia care. Without such a method, Kitwood argued, person-centred care is in danger of remaining a vague aspiration, lacking in empirical foundation. Anxious to ensure that his notion of person-centred care has a demonstrable impact in the real world of dementia care, the burgeoning usage of DCM played a key part in Kitwood's strategy and, although publications on DCM formed a relatively small proportion of Kitwood's prodigious output, the degree of effort invested by the Bradford Group in developing the technique and in training hundreds of practitioners in its use has been large. The fact that the sixth edition of the manual appeared at the beginning of its sixth year in existence is indicative of the attention that has been paid to refining the method.

The catalyst which prompted the initial development of DCM was a request for the Bradford Dementia Group to evaluate a day service for people with dementia (Kitwood, 1994, p22). The group's attempt to incorporate the views of all concerned with the service floundered for want of an established method of assessing the quality of the service from the perspective of the users themselves. No research tool had been developed which would compensate for the impact of memory loss on the person with dementia's ability to make cumulative judgements about their past experiences of the service. In order to fill this vacuum, Kitwood and Kathleen Bredin created an observational method which sought to unearth the nature of care as it is experienced, minute by minute, by the person with dementia. Their labours produced a tool which is gaining widespread acceptance as the leading method currently available for the evaluation of the quality of dementia care.

It was not the intention of the Bradford Group to produce a tool whose primary use would be in research and which would be judged against the criterion of scientific reliability. DCM is a process of developmental evaluation and, as such, needs to be accepted by staff. It requires staff involvement both in discussion of its findings and in planning to meet any areas for improvement that are identified. Thus greater importance is attached to care staff finding its conclusions relevant and useful than to its gaining credibility amongst the academic scientific community. Nonetheless, there are, as mentioned, close conceptual links to Kitwood's theory of dementia and dementia care and he was sufficiently confident in these links to assert that DCM is able both to ascertain how personhood is maintained and to assess whether person-centred care is taking place.

Certainly, the volume of data that DCM produces is impressive and many of those familiar with it in practice find it is able to discern the quality of psychological care and to provide an explanation of the tangible factors that differentiate different levels of quality. It is very much an observation of the process of care as it has an impact upon the person with dementia and it rests upon an assumption that for a group of, say, ten or more people there is a direct relationship between their relative well-being and the quality of the care that they receive.

Whilst it is not my intention here to go into the detailed mechanics of DCM, I will attempt to give a brief outline of its method, which consists of a trained 'mapper', or a team of mappers, each spending a period of some hours observing between five and eight people with dementia each. The mapper uses three coding frames, the first of which relates to the behaviour of the person with dementia. Here the mapper records at five-minute intervals the dominant activity from the 24 categories contained in the Behaviour Category Coding (BCC). There are clear rules for ascertaining which activity amongst the many that can occur in any five-minute time frame should take precedence for recording purposes and also for which of the six bands of well-being and ill-being (the WIB score) should be applied. Over a period of, say, five hours observing five individuals a mapper will have gained some 600 pieces of information which, when analysed, give a clear picture not only of the pattern of (in)activity within the setting but also of the quality of experience of care provided.

The quality of care is also monitored by the two coding frames which relate directly to the behaviour of staff, firstly by recording incidents in which 'personal detractions' (PDs) occur. Personal detractions are instances of the 17 aspects of Malignant Social Psychology which are graded, according to their severity, as mild, moderate, severe or very severe. Their counterpart is chronicled in the more recently developed Positive Event recording in which the mapper notes any episodes of good practice that can be fed back to staff in order to raise awareness and generalise skills being displayed sporadically or by particular staff.

Observation is only carried out in 'public' areas and mappers aim to blend in with the care environment, helping to carry out care tasks when appropriate and being quite open with staff and service users about their presence and their purpose. DCM's success as a developmental tool is closely aligned to the degree to which staff are comfortable with its aims and methods so that a great deal of care is taken in preparing staff for the exercise and in attempting to establish a non-threatening relationship which is not perceived as being akin to an 'inspection' of any kind. The developmental process consists of staff utilising the feedback from the mapping to increase collective awareness of their practice. It is therefore essential that they are not manoeuvred into a position which encourages them to be defensive about current practice and/or dismissive of the results of the exercise. In those areas that Kitwood identified as having eliminated most of the Malignant Social Psychology but then remaining static, this is all the more important, if they are to move on to creating more positively therapeutic psychological environments.

The degree of success achieved by DCM in bringing about genuine and sustained change in the way in which dementia care is delivered is strongly influenced by the way in which it is organised. There are real limitations imposed by the most common arrangements for mapping, in which a trained mapper from outside the organisation is brought in, firstly to map a care environment, and then to meet the staff group to feed back the results (usually contained in a report) and discuss strategies for improvement. The hope is that such meetings will influence the future behaviour of staff, largely as a result of influencing their attitudes to their work, but there is some doubt as to how much can be achieved in this regard with just the one or two meetings that this approach involves. Yet the experience of mapping itself, spending several hours observing the care environment and attempting to take the view of the person with dementia, has an intense impact on one's attitude to care. Therefore a more productive approach might be to encourage the training of teams of staff in order that they may map their own work environment. Such an approach would have to overcome the obvious logistical difficulties and would require a sensitivity to the potential impact on team dynamics. The anecdotal evidence provided by three nursing assistants from Bristol (Packer *et al*, 1996), however, suggests that such an investment could well prove worthwhile.

Another difficulty surrounding the organisation of DCM concerns the control of the information that it yields. The Bradford Group are insistent that DCM should not be used as a tool with which managers 'judge' groups of staff and attempt to introduce changes by utilising the power that accompanies their position in the organisational hierarchy. The emphasis is very much on a collaborative partnership between those carrying out the mapping and the staff group, with management being kept at something of an 'arms length', perhaps not even being allowed to view the results at all. While this approach may be justifiable in terms of the need to gain the trust and acceptance of the staff group, it can detract from their ability to gain access to any resources (in terms of training, extra staff or input from other disciplines) which are identified as necessary to secure a lasting improvement. Few managers would be willing to agree to a claim for extra resources from a care environment while being denied access to the data on which such a claim is based.

With the DCM method now in its seventh edition, the number of trained mappers runs well into the hundreds and a smaller group of 'master' practitioners have been using the method for a considerable time, enabling them to participate in and influence its continual refinement. While the method focuses on the processes of care as opposed to the organisational features of the care environment, recent work (for example, Bredin *et al*, 1995; Perrin, 1997) reveals potential implications for the way that care is structured. The future may well reveal that DCM has as much to say to those holding influence over the way services are developed as it currently says to those who provide the actual care.

Some Reflections and Comments

It was noted at the beginning of this chapter that there appears to be an almost logical progression to Kitwood's work. Viewed retrospectively, it can give the impression of having been a grand project, gradually revealing itself as the conclusions of one phase of his writing and activity flow into the themes and concerns of the next. This perception is misleading, however, to the extent that it fails to take into account the difficult, sometimes hostile, environment in which his ideas were being generated. Kitwood's earliest expression of his theory of dementia was seen by many as threatening the accepted view of the psychiatric profession and also that of carers' organisations, notably the Alzheimer's Disease Society, which had made a heavy investment in generating publicity based on the standard paradigm view of dementia. We should try to understand Kitwood's work, then, not only in relation to its inner dynamic but also in relation to the historical situation of dementia care at the time it was being produced. Just as our understanding of the writings of political theorists can be aided by an awareness of the political context in which they were active, so an appreciation of the situation of dementia care in the late 1980s and early 1990s helps us to grasp some of the emphasis and preoccupations in Kitwood's work. If certain points in his earlier work now seem to be rather overstated, this is largely symptomatic of the extent of the divide that existed between his, still novel, position and that of mainstream thought on dementia at the time. The fact that this gulf has been bridged in more recent years largely as a result of a change in the direction of the mainstream is testament to the degree of success that he achieved.

This section aims to draw out some of the issues that seem to have been at the heart of the controversies that Kitwood provoked. I believe, as the reader will already have gathered, that many of these controversies were both useful and necessary, and I have tried to indicate my support for particular positions as they arose in the text. This final section will be focusing more on areas that are still ripe for disagreement and for further debate.

The Medicalisation of Alzheimer's Disease
In his first article on dementia Kitwood (1987a) is concerned with the way dementia is viewed, especially since 'the psychological afflictions of old age have been reclassified, and the majority of cases of dementia are claimed to be due to Alzheimer's Disease' (p81). The reader is left with little doubt as to Kitwood's cynicism regarding this claim. This article, which was shortly to be followed by an incisive critique of the research evidence behind the claim, examines the standard paradigm view of Alzheimer's Disease implicit in Marion Roach's account of her mother's dementia (Roach, 1985). It left Kitwood 'disturbed by the account as ideology, as a reflection of the heartless common sense of the taken-for-granted world of late capitalism' (Kitwood, 1987a, p82).

Throughout this article and subsequent early texts, Kitwood consistently equated the acceptance, or rejection, of the standard paradigm view with an acceptance, or rejection of a political (in its broadest sense) position. The standard paradigm view is seen as being in accordance with the aims and values of, variously, industrial and/or capitalist societies. Indeed, Roach's story of her mother's dementia is summarised as 'a naive and exceptionally open description of the dehumanising character of the everyday life of late capitalism, within which a woman was psychologically destroyed' (ibid.). The reader is never enlightened, however, as to what the nature of the relationship between capitalism and our understanding of dementia, or between capitalism and an individual's experience of dementia, might be.

Kitwood's more recent writings contain no references to 'capitalism', either as a factor in promoting a particular view of dementia or as a necessary component to understanding its aetiology. The 'Alzheimerisation' of dementia is now explained as a pragmatic decision, designed to attract more funding in the USA in the mid-1980s (Kitwood, 1997a, p22) and, while the Malignant Social Psychology is explained to some extent as an instance of Fromm's 'pathology of normality', there is no attempt to establish such direct links between the nature of society and the course of an individual's dementia. Certainly, there are connections between mental health problems and the political, economic and social context in which they occur, but it should be acknowledged that the early Kitwood was unable to give to this aspect the attention it deserves. The question of how the social, economic and political context affects either the belief system of a particular sub-group or the mental condition of an individual is, of course, highly complex and is itself explicable only in relation to its own historical context. The predicament of the individual trapped in mind-numbingly boring factory work differs from that of the unemployed member of a destroyed ex-mining community, which differs from that of the recently redundant executive, which differs again from that of the stressed-out nurse. Our understanding of any of these is not enhanced by simplistic, imprecise generalisations about 'capitalism' or 'industrialism', however much they may appear to serve social psychology's ambition to relate the individual and the interpersonal to sociostructural phenomena. Indeed, such references actually carry a determinism of their own, which has been refuted, at least in part, by Kitwood's own success. Acceptance of the standard paradigm in Britain has waned, owing in no small measure to his efforts, during a period in which 'capitalism' and 'industrialism' have, if anything, been strengthened.

The Critique of the Standard Paradigm

Kitwood was clearly better equipped than Naomi Feil before him in making a coherent attempt to challenge the commonly accepted view of dementia as a purely organic mental illness. He was able to expose both the rather weak empirical evidence that supported it and its shaky theoretical foundations. His success in revealing the extreme reductionism and crude materialism that make up such foundations has left fewer people willing to come forward as unconditional exponents of the standard paradigm. Indeed, it is questionable how much overt support was ever available for a paradigm that had become more of an unspoken premise, an assumption that cast a shadow over a generation of professionals involved with dementia and brought them to speak and act as if it were true. Its hegemonic position at the centre of orthodox opinion was under threat from the moment that the extreme reductionism that constitutes its own philosophical premise was exposed. For no phenomena involving 'meaning' can ever be fully accounted for in wholly materialistic terms, that is in terms of physical phenomena alone. This is as true of something such as a book as it is of the human mind. Imagine, for a moment, a pure reductionist — restricted to using material terms alone — attempting to give a full account of this book. While they may, in theory, be able to describe the position of each and every one of the smallest known particles that constitute the physical object you are now looking at, they would not have access to any of the terminology required to explain what a single sentence means. Meaning is not a physical category. Similarly psychology, which must deal with phenomena like meaning and perceptions, can never be reduced, or translated, purely into terms used by the neurosciences. This is not to deny the role of the neurosciences, it is merely to acknowledge that it has its limits and that these are reached at the point at which we begin to deal with meaning.

When Kitwood began to examine the question of dementia, the standard paradigm view prevailed, medical hegemony was unchallenged and the quality of dementia care left, with only a few notable exceptions, much to be desired. Such circumstances make it understandable, therefore, that Kitwood should see the association between these three aspects as being particularly strong. In his list of 'differences between the old and new cultures of dementia care' (Kitwood, 1995, p8) he links the standard paradigm, as the old culture's 'general view of dementia', with the avoidance of psychological considerations in the old culture's notion of 'what caring involves'. He sees caregivers that adopt a more holistic view of the person with dementia as engaging in a kind of 'doublethink':

> The 'standard paradigm' is what they officially believe, on the basis of what they have read or been taught. But they also hold, unofficially and intuitively, a more optimistic and less deterministic theory about dementia; usually they cannot articulate it clearly, but it is this that informs their practice.
> (Kitwood, 1990a, p179–180)

My view is that there was rather more to this tendency than 'doublethink' and that the actual historical relationship between the standard paradigm and the culture of care is less interlinked than Kitwood was led to believe. While there is undoubtedly a conceptual connection between the standard paradigm and impoverished psychological care, the actual historical relationship between the two has been more ambiguous. As Bob Woods and others have pointed out (Woods, 1995; Bleathman & Morton, 1994) psychological approaches to dementia care can be traced back to the 1950s and although the earliest authors on the effects of stimulation (Cosin *et al*, 1958) and Reality Orientation (Taulbee & Folsom, 1966) may have been primarily concerned with cognition, the growth in the use of reminiscence with people with dementia actually coincided with standard paradigm's ascendancy, following the research trials of the late 1960s and early 1970s. Although there is no doubt that the general standards of psychological care of people with dementia would be viewed as unacceptable by today's standards, from the late 1950s onwards there was a widespread acknowledgement amongst the relevant professions that psychological approaches could have a real impact on dementia. The problem was that the preoccupation with the cognitive aspects of the condition led to a long period of over-reliance on one approach, Reality Orientation, which left caregivers at a loss in their attempts to address the emotional needs of people with dementia. It was this vacuum that created the conditions leading to the great surge of interest that met the emergence of Validation and Resolution Therapy. Caregivers were not looking for a new theoretical framework for understanding dementia so much as guidance in easing the distress which accompanied the condition — guidance which RO was patently unable to provide.

The complexity of the development of dementia care in Britain suggests that the dichotomy of 'old' and 'new' cultures of care is not a particularly helpful way of achieving an understanding of the way in which care has developed and, therefore, of the direction that we might expect it to take in the future. Proposing such a dichotomy might serve as a rallying call, or act as a caricature, drawn to facilitate the expression of an aspiration. The danger is that it is likely to be taken too literally, tempting us to define characteristics of old and new cultures and to judge progress solely as a function of this kind of cultural change. The undoubted advances of recent years were largely grounded in the experience of caregivers, a section of whom revolted against the continuing imposition of a predominantly cognitive perspective and demanded that the wider, human aspects of their roles be addressed. The standard paradigm may have served to a few as a disincentive to pursue the possibilities for developing dementia care, but the general improvement has probably been driven by those who still hold a 'soft' version, accepting a stronger association between neuropathology and symptoms than Kitwood would. The general advance should also be viewed in the light of parallel advances in other areas of mental health care, especially Learning Disabilities, and partially as a consequence of the influx of talent drawn to old age psychiatry by the opportunities for career progression that, by the mid-1980s, demographic factors had begun to promise.

I have dwelt upon the issue of the relationship between the theoretical framework used to make sense of dementia and the quality of care because there is a danger that one might infer from Kitwood's work that the latter is in some way contingent upon the former. I would argue that our perception of the implications of any mental health problem is reframed by the simple act of increasing our awareness of that which we have in common (our 'humanity') and reducing the significance we attach to that which differentiates us (the illness). This line, which also runs through Kitwood's work on personhood, is a key element of the person-centred approach in that it draws us away from the cognitive and towards the relational. It also removes the risk of the person-centred approach being undermined by future research, which may establish stronger links between neuropathology and dementia, or of becoming dependent on Kitwood's own theoretical framework.

Is there a Dialectic of Dementia?

As pointed out earlier, after rejecting the standard paradigm view of dementia, Kitwood hypothesised that the dementing process consists of a dialectical interplay between neurological factors and the Malignant Social Psychology (Kitwood, 1990a). More recently he stated that 'the lack of well-functioning interneuronal circuitry' which causes dementia has:

> background causes [which] may be related to a pathology that has its own dynamic; but also, they may be related to psychological factors, which initially have their counterpart in neurochemistry and, eventually, in the way brain circuitry fails to develop, or is destroyed. We can thus view the process of dementia as involving a continuing interplay between those factors that pertain to neuropathology per se and those which are social–psychological. (Kitwood, 1997a, p50)

Kitwood appears to have gone some way beyond what the current evidence allows us to say with any reasonable degree of certainty here. Having argued convincingly that the correlation between the clinical appearance of dementia and neurological impairment is too weak to justify the standard paradigm assertion, 'SD = NI', Kitwood comes forward with a missing factor 'MSP' and suggests that now we have a fuller explanation, 'SD = MSP + NI'. But there is, of course, even less evidence to link Malignant Social Psychology with dementia than there is to link Neurological Impairment with dementia. In terms of the above passage, there is currently no evidence to support the claim that 'negative' psychological factors actually do influence the way brain circuitry 'fails to develop or is destroyed'. It is one thing to acknowledge that each psychological event has its neurological counterpart but quite another to claim that we know what that counterpart is. In thus implying such a claim, Kitwood shares a bond with Naomi Feil and he runs a similar risk of alienating opinion which would otherwise be receptive to his insights.

Kitwood had a tendency to express ideas as theoretical possibilities and then proceed to build arguments that are conditional upon their acceptance. The above passage is a good example, as in the first sentence psychological factors 'may' be related to the causes of the dementia, yet by the second sentence we are viewing dementia as if they are. Here is another example:

Some changes in brain structure may indeed be caused by a process that has its own (non-psychological) dynamic; other changes, however, are consequent upon experience. A malignant social–psychological environment might retard the development of new circuitry, or even accelerate the advance of neurological degeneration.
(Ibid.)

It is true that MSP might have these neurological effects, but it is equally true that they might not or, for that matter, that they might have the opposite effects. Our knowledge regarding the nature of the relationship between the psychological and the neurological in this regard is so limited that we are reduced to conjecture and, currently, only an act of faith can sustain the belief that the counterpart of a negative psychological event is a (significantly) negative neurological event. As we might expect, Kitwood was well aware of this shortcoming, and of the need to remedy it by researching the long-term neurological effects of good care.

When considering the equations that Kitwood uses to describe the process of dementia (SD = NI + MSP, SD = P + B + H + NI + SP) there are three related questions which remain unanswered.

1 What is the causal weight of each of these factors, and how can we know it is sufficient in each case to be included as a causal factor? With regards to the more recently developed equation, $SD = P + B + H + NI + SP$, how do we know that the psychological aspects (P, B and SP) have any more causal weight than they do in, say, diabetes or any other physical condition?

2 Similarly, what evidence is there that the dynamic of NI (the manner in which it develops) is influenced by either P, B or SP?

3 Are the psychological factors P, B and SP included as factors which cause a dementing illness, or as factors which influence the way a person responds when they have a dementing illness?

This third question leads us into a key area of Kitwood's thinking on dementia. It is possible to read two possible accounts of dementia, differentiated by the degree of influence they are prepared to concede to neuropathology. They can be described as a 'harder' and a 'softer' version. The harder version contends that it was an error to classify dementia as an organic mental illness, as distinct from functional mental illnesses such as psychoses and depression. In fact, dementia should be seen as a kind of psychosis. As we age, our brains degenerate to the extent that a mental illness in old age (which in younger life would not appear to cause significant structural damage) is set in a much more fragile neurological environment, increasing the prospect of damage. On post-mortem such damage is observed and assumed to be the cause of dementia, but in reality this damage may be epiphenomenal. Thus we all have a threshold for developing dementia, which decreases with age, and our susceptibility is dependent upon the pre-existing condition of our brain and upon the extent of 'dementogenic' factors, especially stress, that we encounter. Once neurological damage has occurred, the extent of future damage will continue to be a function of our psychosocial environment which, if of suitable quality, may even provide for some neurological improvement.

The softer version concedes that there is real neuropathology — operating largely to its own dynamic — at work in dementia, and that this affects cognitive functioning. In the past, however, it has been mistakenly assumed that the decline in many other aspects associated with dementia is a 'symptom' of the disease. It is likely that whereas neurological impairment may cause the cognitive decline (memory problems, communication difficulties, disorientation, some degree of dyspraxia, and so on) other factors, especially mood disturbance, personality change, behavioural problems and some of the loss of skills, are in fact a function of the psychosocial environment, especially the quality of care.

The Malignant Social Psychology

Much of Kitwood's appeal to those involved in dementia care is founded on his description of the Malignant Social Psychology, a description instantly recognised by many, yet previously stated by none. Nobody has drawn a more perceptive and incisive picture of the everyday world of the person with dementia and their carers, or helped so many carers to redefine what is unacceptable in dementia care by pointing out the damage done by behaviour that previously went both unidentified and unchallenged.

This is, of course, enormously to Kitwood's credit and his achievement should be borne in mind when considering any attempt at criticism of the theoretical cogency of his position, which probably results from the previously observed shift in his use of the term 'social psychology'. In his early writings on dementia Kitwood began to use the term 'social psychology' to denote not an academic discipline but rather a 'thing', which could be judged as healthy or otherwise. Kitwood used 'the malignant social psychology' as a kind of shorthand for 'the characteristic unhelpful actions and attitudes of those surrounding the person with dementia', and acknowledged that being on the receiving end of such actions and attitudes is not unique to dementia sufferers. Such shorthand has its uses, but it is not necessarily the case that such reification actually helps our understanding. As has been outlined elsewhere (Morton, 1997) it appears that, having posited the existence of an entity, MSP, Kitwood developed an explanation for its existence that underestimated the role played by differentials in power. Studying the social psychology of groups that are marginalised or persecuted in society, or of those that occupy the lower positions in hierarchies (usually at work), reveals a 'malignancy' that is a function of their relative lack of power and control in shaping their social–psychological environment.

Kitwood acknowledged that being on the receiving end of MSP is not unique to dementia sufferers, but any attempt to address the problems identified by the concept of MSP perhaps needs to be grounded in an account of the power relationships between those involved, and we need to be both creative and realistic in assessing how these might be reformed. The issue of power is not absent from Kitwood's work, but it has tended to be considered more in relation to organisational structure and style as opposed to the relationship between service providers and users.

Dementia Care Mapping
It is also worth looking briefly at the relationship between Dementia Care Mapping (DCM) and Kitwood's understanding of dementia as it is sometimes assumed, mistakenly, that there is a strong theoretical link between the two. This assumption usually contends that DCM actually measures the Malignant Social Psychology and is able to demonstrate correlation between MSP and relative well-being. We need to be clear, therefore, that DCM seeks to measure what people with dementia are doing over a period of time and also their relative well-being. Its data, therefore, might be used to demonstrate correlation between the variety of types of activity available and apparent well-being, for example. What it cannot do, however, is provide empirical support for Kitwood's model of dementia, as the method actually rests upon the assumptions that are explicit in the model itself. Thus, as we saw earlier, DCM assumes that there is a link between well-being and quality of care but it does not seek to quantify quality of care in relation to Kitwood's key construct, the Malignant Social Psychology. Although DCM comments upon episodes of MSP, in the form of personal detractions, it does not relate these either to (transient) relative well-being or to any longer-term aspects of the observed person's mental health. This is not to detract from DCM's position as the most advanced evaluative tool currently available to dementia care; rather, it is to claim that DCM could have been developed by someone with quite different views on the nature of dementia. Thus the conceptual link between Dementia Care Mapping and Kitwood's theory of dementia is actually rather weak, and this has been a source of some frustration to those who would have preferred

to see the Bradford Group operationalising the constructs in Kitwood's model of dementia and subjecting it to rigorous research.

Was Kitwood Person-Centred?

Such is the extent of his influence that, in Britain at least, those involved in dementia care who espouse the need for a 'person-centred' approach are usually referring to the sense in which it was used by Tom Kitwood, as opposed to advocating the principles developed by Carl Rogers. If we take the term 'person-centred' as being synonymous with 'Rogerian' then we would have to say that, whilst Rogers has undoubtedly influenced Kitwood, he is just one of many sources of inspiration behind the latter's theory of dementia care. We have seen how ideas derived from psychotherapy play a major role in Kitwood's thinking and how they are joined by concepts derived from social psychology, political theory and ethics. Indeed, he has spoken of person-centred care as combining ethics, in the form of respect for persons, and social psychology which provides the understanding necessary to put the ethic into practice.

Even within the field of psychotherapy, there are a host of differing influences on Kitwood's understanding of the human condition, as he acknowledged in one of his earliest articles: 'I have found myself becoming, at different times, a disciple of Freud, Klein, Jung, Bern, Rogers, Perls and several others in my own attempts to make sense of the dementing experience' (Kitwood, 1990c, p48).

The multiplicity of meanings that have become attached to the term 'person-centred' were discussed at the beginning of this book. Kitwood's usage in describing his own approach to care is closer to the 'everyday' meaning outlined there, in that the 'person' can be said to be at the centre of one's considerations. Notwithstanding the evidence of a strong Rogerian influence on Kitwood, there is much in his outlook that a Rogerian Person-Centred Therapist would rule outside a definition of their own work. While it may, in the end, be just a question of semantics, perhaps the (somewhat clumsy) term 'personhood enhancing' would serve Kitwood's purpose better, in that it both carries an indication of the essential social psychological component of his thought and avoids the confusion which is inherent in two approaches using the same term to describe what are in many respects quite different things. Such confusion, and much unnecessary debate, may well occur when an approach which is 'person-centred' in the purely Rogerian sense arrives on the scene of dementia care, as seems more than likely with the emergence of Pre-Therapy.

Spring Mount: Person-Centred Dementia Care in Action

It is one of history's happier, and more remarkable, coincidences that Tom Kitwood conducted his earliest theoretical excursions into dementia and dementia care while working in the same northern city as two individuals who had already decided to act on their own convictions and develop a radically different approach to the care of people with dementia.

Prior to their opening Spring Mount Residential Home in Bradford in 1987, Janet Bell and Iain McGregor were employed by the local NHS community psychiatric service for the elderly, working as a community psychiatric nurse and psychiatric social worker, respectively. Both had become disillusioned by the poverty of the service that was offered to people with dementia, epitomised by its reliance on the use of neuroleptic medication to deal with behavioural problems which, in Bell and McGregor's eyes, sprang directly from the inadequacies of care. One of their earliest decisions upon resolving to provide an alternative approach to residential care was to eliminate the use of tranquillising medication for residents. This they did in co-operation with the local family doctor, initially by graduated withdrawal, before concluding that it was more effective to stop neuroleptics altogether as soon as people moved into Spring Mount. Significant initial hostility from some local health professionals having been overcome, the experience of witnessing the effects of their policy on over one hundred people who have been residents leaves the pair convinced that this original judgement was correct: 'We do not believe that anyone who has dementia is ever helped by the use of tranquillisers, or indeed by sedation of any sort' (Bell & McGregor, 1994, p15). Their early determination to eradicate reliance on unnecessary medication has been complemented by an ethos which aims to break free from what they see as a cluster of unhelpful myths about dementia. In a series of three articles Bell and McGregor have identified a 'series of misunderstandings about what dementia actually does to people' (ibid). Such myths include the following:

- dementia makes people violent and aggressive;
- dementia destroys personality;
- tranquillisers are necessary to control the behaviour of people with dementia;
- dementia makes people less sociable and unable to enjoy new relationships;
- dementia makes people sexually disinhibited and unable to understand sexual responsibility;
- people with dementia are not able to make a positive contribution to group living;
- people with dementia are unable to exercise self-determination and make choices for themselves;
- people with dementia wander aimlessly;
- people with dementia lose the ability for new learning.
  (Adapted from Bell & McGregor, 1994; McGregor & Bell, 1994a, 1994b)

The prevalence, and ingrained nature, of these beliefs amongst those involved in the care of people with dementia has meant that Spring Mount has largely excluded applicants with previous experience in the field when recruiting care staff. Its proprietors have felt that the habits of relying on medication to control behaviour, the need to keep a 'professional' distance from residents, the propensity to develop institutionalised working patterns and the tendency to hold on to beliefs such as those listed above all militate against 'experienced' staff being able to realise the philosophy of Spring Mount in practice.

The resulting care environment at Spring Mount has echoes of the principles of social role valorisation (Wolfensberger, 1983), the social model of disability (for example, Oliver, 1983; Makin, 1995) and the therapeutic community movement (Jones, 1953). While it acknowledges that disabilities, especially in the areas of memory, communication and practical skills, are very real and require compensatory action by staff, residents remain in control of their social situation and in charge of how they spend their day. Staff do not interfere in interactions between residents, even if they become hostile, nor do they exert control over residents with aspects of their daily routine, such as bed-times. Staff are encouraged to develop deeper interpersonal relationships with residents, acknowledging their losses and facilitating adjustment, exploration and development.

While acknowledging the presence of real cognitive deficits in their residents, Bell and McGregor argue, as the list of 'myths' above indicates, that many of the other 'symptoms' associated with dementia are actually the result of secondary factors which are provoked by the onset of cognitive impairment. Chief amongst such 'symptoms' are changes in personality, behaviour and mood and the loss of social skills, all of which are often seen as direct consequences of neuropathology. The lesson that Bell and McGregor have drawn from their experience is that such changes are more likely to be indicative of social withdrawal, a response to the experience of dementia that is exacerbated by the attitudes that it induces in others. Such withdrawal is often compounded by the effects of sedation. They cite numerous occasions on which relatives of Spring Mount residents comment how their loved ones are 'back to their old selves' or have 'got their own personality back'. Bell and McGregor interpret comments such as this as evidence that these personalities were never in fact lost, they were simply buried, or masked, by poor care environments and by medication, so that when these factors were removed the previous personality 'resurfaced'.

Access to the unique care environment of Spring Mount, and to the ideas of its proprietors, helped to confirm Kitwood's belief in the potential for an understanding of dementia that was rooted in social psychology. It provided him with a living example of the kind of 'relative well-being' that was achievable in dementia — a notion which was to become integral to the development of Dementia Care Mapping. Although the chord struck by Kitwood's ideas led to his taking much of the credit for the transformation of the way in which dementia care is perceived in Britain, it would be a mistake to underestimate the contribution that Bell and McGregor made to the development of those ideas by their demonstration that good quality dementia care can achieve far more than was previously imagined.

CHAPTER 5

The Relevance of Prouty's Pre-Therapy to Dementia Care

Dion van Werde & Ian Morton

Introduction

The founder of Pre-Therapy, Garry Prouty, has expanded the scope of 'classical' Rogerian therapy to include work with people whose functioning is impaired. In doing so, he has ensured that considerations regarding the quality of the relationship between client and caregiver, and regarding the experiential world of the client, are central to the development of a way of working with, and of understanding, people who show some degree of 'problematic' behaviour. Such an approach is, both in its theory and its practice, opposed to the 'symptom-centredness' that characterises strictly biological or behavioural accounts and it is expressed in a way of working that is truly 'person-centred'. Pre-Therapy entails a holistic view that looks beyond visible behaviour, seeking a fresh way of tuning into people with impairment and a way of working that is characterised by existential depth. It should be added at this early stage, however, that this experiential viewpoint does not entail an abandonment of the goals of promoting functioning in everyday life, or of setting the limits that are required for social living.

In this initial look at the potential relevance of Pre-Therapy for work with people who have dementia, we shall introduce the key constructs of Prouty's work before focusing on the reasoning behind the practice of Pre-Therapy, rather than on the practice itself. There is, as yet, no documentation of the use of Pre-Therapy with people with dementia and during these very early stages of investigation into its potential application to this client population, we believe that an understanding of the evolution of the rationale of Pre-Therapy is particularly important. Only when such an understanding is achieved, and the practical skills required for Pre-Therapy are mastered, will we be in a position to fully explore this field in practice.

Each of the approaches described in the preceding three chapters represents, in varying degrees, the growing influence of the person-centred tradition on dementia care. Validation and Resolution Therapy are both examples of attempts by professionals working in the field of dementia to 'import' aspects of the person-centred approach into their understanding of the condition and to apply its principles to the practice of care. Tom Kitwood, on the other hand, began his work on dementia having already gained a well-developed grounding in humanistic psychology. The subject of this chapter, Pre-Therapy, can be seen as a move from within the person-centred movement to 'export' its principles and practice beyond the boundaries of its traditional client population and setting, hence the title of Prouty's book (1994) on Pre-Therapy: *Theoretical Evolutions in Person-Centered/Experiential Therapy*. Exponents have, thus far, largely concentrated their endeavours on working with people diagnosed as 'psychotic', with those who have come to be known in Britain as having 'learning disabilities' (Peters, 1992; Pörtner, 1996) and with individuals who have attracted both labels. The use of Pre-Therapy with people with dementia is, therefore, largely unexplored and it is our hope that readers will agree that such an exploration is rich in potential.

This chapter, which seeks to promote the potential suitability of Pre-Therapy for working with people with dementia is the result of a cross-fertilisation of ideas between a clinical practitioner working in the field of dementia care and a skilled Pre-Therapist who has witnessed the relevance of Pre-Therapy through years of practice with psychotic people in individual therapy, through the development of the concept of the therapeutic contact milieu (see, for example, Prouty *et al*, 1998) and also through his personal experience of being with a relative who suffered from a brain dysfunction. We have not sought to produce a manual of what to do and when and how to do it, but rather to take you by the hand and guide you towards the clinical relevance of Pre-Therapy as applied to people with dementia.

We begin by introducing Garry Prouty and his highly original contribution to the evolution of person-centred psychotherapy. We will illustrate his theory with brief examples from practice with psychotic clients before considering some key notions which will enable us to formulate some possibilities for individual practice with dementing people.

Although Pre-Therapy has now become an established part of the person-centred culture in Europe and North America, its theory and practice were developed over many years by its founder, Garry Prouty. Prouty describes his own mother as having been 'psychotic' and his brother as 'mentally retarded' and 'distressed' (Prouty et al, 1998, p17). His early therapeutic work in the mid-1960s involved work on 'back wards' with chronic schizophrenics under the supervision of Eugene Gendlin, whose emphasis on the role of experiencing is acknowledged as influencing the shift of person-centred thought away from the purely relationship theory developed by Rogers in the 1940s and 1950s (Prouty, 1994, pp15–16).

In the decade that followed, Prouty's work with this client group drew his attention to the first of what Rogers (1957b) described as the six 'Necessary and Sufficient Conditions for Constructive Personality Change':

For constructive personality change to occur, it is necessary that these conditions exist and continue over a period of time:

1. Two persons are in psychological contact.
2. The first, whom we shall term the client, is in a stage of incongruence, being vulnerable or anxious.
3. The second person, whom we shall call the therapist, is congruent or integrated in the relationship.
4. The therapist experiences unconditional positive regard for the client.

5. The therapist experiences an empathic understanding of the client's internal frame of reference and endeavours to communicate this experience to the client.
6. The communication to the client of the therapist's empathic understanding and unconditional positive regard is to a minimal degree achieved.

No other conditions are necessary. If these six conditions exist, and continue over a period of time, this is sufficient. The process of constructive personality change will follow.

Whereas Rogers took the first condition 'psychological contact' as given, Prouty (1994, p36) realised that it can, in fact, be problematic, as: 'Many clients are not fully capable of maintaining therapeutic relationships, as is the case with the schizophrenic and retarded/psychotic populations.'

Pre-Therapy, then, was initially conceived as a method of facilitating psychological contact, as a 'precondition' of therapy. Its function is to enable the client to move from the 'pre-relationship' stage into a therapeutic relationship in which the other five conditions can be met. Experience has shown, however, that the goal of entering psychotherapy in the traditional person-centred sense is often unrealistic. As a result, attention has increasingly been given to the lack of contact between the individual and her/his experience, working with the 'pre-experiential' functioning of the client.

Whilst it is too early yet to see the full historical significance of Pre-Therapy, its aim is to open up areas of mental health that have remained largely neglected by person-centred theorists and practitioners since the difficulties Rogers encountered in his contact with mainstream psychiatry at Wisconsin (Kirschenbaum, 1980, pp275–318). In confronting the historical limitations of the role of the Person-Centred Therapist, of the setting of therapy and of the nature of its client populations, Pre-Therapy challenges the uneasy boundaries that have separated the spheres of influence of psychiatry and Person-Centred Therapy. As it can be argued that such boundaries have served neither side well, such a challenge will be welcomed by many.

Prouty's Pre-Therapy

Pre-Therapy is a theory of 'contact' which seeks to address issues that are implicit in the first of Rogers' six conditions. The theory contains three central constructs: contact functions, contact reflections and contact behaviours.

Contact Functions

The concept of contact functions is derived from Fritz Perls' concept of 'contact as an ego function' (Prouty, 1994, p40). It is the contact functions that are held to be impaired in psychosis and/or brain damage and that Pre-Therapy hopes to restore. There are three fields of contact:

1 'reality contact', which refers to our contact with, and our awareness of, the world — people, places, objects and events;
2 'affective contact', which concerns our awareness of how we respond to the world. It refers to our relationship with our self and our experience, our moods, feelings and emotions;
3 'communicative contact', which consists of our attempts to convey our perception of reality and affect to others. It is a precondition to our forming psychological contact with others and primarily involves the use of socially understandable language.

The impairment of contact functions renders the individual, to a greater or lesser extent, either unable to locate themselves as the locus of their own experience and process or unable to communicate that experience to others. Psychosis is seen as an idiosyncratic loss of contact with experience.

Contact Reflections

'Contact reflections' are the techniques which the therapist uses to build and/or strengthen contact functions. Reflection as a technique was first developed by Otto Rank, the Austrian psychologist and psychotherapist who was one of Freud's earliest students. After his break from Freud in the 1930s, he began using reflection of his client's statements, primarily as a means of clarifying his own understanding of his client's view of the world. Despite his psychoanalytic credentials, Rank is acknowledged (for example, Thorne, 1992, pp58–59) as a forerunner of the person-centred approach in that he advocated a less directive role for the therapist and emphasised the therapeutic role of the relationship between client and therapist.

The influence of Rank on the direction of Rogers' early thinking evolved into the latter using reflection as a means by which the therapist offers a relationship to the client. Reflection became a kind of sensitive and empathic responsiveness, enabling the therapist to check the accuracy of their appreciation of the client's frame of reference while conveying the therapist's empathy to the client.

Eugene Gendlin, an early associate of Rogers, directed attention towards the experiencing process which takes place during therapy, conceiving therapeutic change as a bodily felt experience. Prouty (1976, p1) sums up the role of reflection as conceived by Gendlin, his former supervisor, thus: 'Stated simply, reflection intensifies inner feeling to the point that an experiencing process is initiated – bringing deeper feeling to the foreground, i.e. therapeutic movement.' In Pre-Therapy the role of reflection owes as much to Gendlin's work as it does to that of Rogers. The notion that feelings can be present, but only potentially experienced (that is, that they can be 'Pre-Experiential') leads to the use of reflection in order to enable the initiation of an experiencing process. Those who are unable to maintain psychological contact — as a result of either psychosocial or organic factors — are seen as being 'unable to experience their feelings with directness or clarity' (ibid.).

The practice of Pre-Therapy consists of the application of four 'contact reflections' and one principle which aim to strengthen the client's contact functions.

Situational Reflections

Situational reflections (SR) are used to strengthen reality contact, contact with the world, especially with regard to the client's immediate physical environment and perceptual field: for example, 'The birds are singing', 'The table is between us', 'The sky is blue', 'clock', 'bed'.

Facial Reflections

Facial reflections (FR) are used to enhance affective contact, contact with the self, by reflecting the feelings that appear to be shown by the client's face: 'Your eyes look sad', 'You look scared', 'You smile', 'Willy looks happy'.

Word-for-Word Reflections

Word-for-word reflections (WWR) are the reflection of coherent communication or meaningful sounds which seek to support communicative contact, or contact with others. The aim is to enable the client to experience themselves as one who communicates. The therapist repeats the coherent utterances of the client. For example:

Client:	I really am scared.
Therapist:	You really are scared.
Client:	Bah!
Therapist:	Bah!
Client:	My head is stone.
Therapist:	My head is stone.
Client:	Pft … bed … king …
Therapist:	Bed.'

Body Reflections

Body reflections (BR) can consist either of: 'an empathic body duplication', in which the therapist mirrors the posture or movements of the client or of a verbal description of the client's position, posture or movements: for example, 'Willy is making a circle with his hands', 'You are sitting cross-legged.', 'Your hand is covering your eyes', 'You are rocking', the client stands in front of the mirror and points at it, whereupon the therapist does the same.

The Reiterative Principle

The contact reflections are supported by the Reiterative Principle (RP), which involves the repetition of earlier reflections that have made contact, evidenced by their eliciting contact behaviours: 'Repeating the psychological contact maximises the opportunity to develop a relationship or to facilitate Experiencing' (Prouty, 1994, p39). For example: 'You pointed, I pointed and you smiled', 'I said "bed" and you stopped rocking.'

Thus the 'techniques' of Pre-Therapy are relatively simple. The real art, however, consists of using them in practice in a way which may benefit clients whose inner world is fragmented and chaotic. In practice, the art of Pre-Therapy is non-directive, in that it follows the process of the client, being directed by the client's actions and expressions. It does not involve interpretation of the client's behaviour. Prouty is clear, however, that the kind of empathy that may be present in the relationship between a therapist and a client who is capable of psychological contact should not be expected in Pre-Therapy. In relation to psychosis, he states: 'The therapist does not know the client's frame of reference' (ibid., p49).

Pre-Therapy does, however, require a heightened sensitivity in the therapist, described by Prouty as 'empathic contact', to:

- the client's effort at developing coherent experience and expression,
- the concrete particularity of behavioural expression,
- the lived experience (of the psychosis, for instance),
- temporal and spatial experience, and
- the appropriate tempo for contact.

Contact Behaviours
The third central construct in Pre-Therapy theory is the means by which improvement in contact functioning can be measured, which Prouty terms 'contact behaviours'. Such behaviours express the client's contact with reality and with their own experiences as well as the capacity to communicate these. In accounting for the increase in contact behaviours in clients of Pre-Therapy, Prouty posits the existence of a 'Pre-Expressive self' which reveals itself through behaviour labelled as psychotic, regressed or autistic. Increases in contact behaviour can be seen as a movement from the pre-expressive to the expressive self.

Prouty cites the example of his own 'mentally retarded' brother, Robert, who reacted to the twelve-year-old Garry's speculating with a friend about whether he could understand anything they said by uttering: 'Garry, you know I do.' This 'thunderbolt' came from someone who had never previously shown any understanding of speech and who, after this comment was made, promptly retreated into his inner world. Prouty produces other accounts of similar instances to support his claim that 'bizarre' speech and behaviour of the psychotic individual is best understood, not in terms of pathology, but rather as being pre-expressive. Thus much psychotic speech actually makes some sort of sense, a sense which is often discernible in the light of increased information about the client's personal history or as more detail of their current phenomenological world is disclosed.

Dealing with Pre-Expressive and 'Grey-Zone' Functioning

Pre-Therapists learn to become aware of the relevance of concrete speech and behaviour and to realise that this is the only 'given' in encounters with people with impaired functioning. Contact with such people is achieved by the use of the formulated Pre-Therapy reflections. For the Pre-Therapist, this is the only way of genuinely reaching the other in a truly human and holistic way, without imposing on the other's personal psychological space. This approach leaves the client with the space they require for the process of attempting to repossess the contents of their own thoughts, their emotions and their efforts to form relationships.

In Prouty's descriptions of his work, he refers to pre-expressive functioning as opposed to expressive, congruent functioning. In the latter case, contact with people, places, events and things (Reality Contact), with emotional functioning (Affective Contact) and with other people (Communicative Contact) is given. The restoration of these contact functions in pre-expressive functioning is the goal of Pre-Therapy. The therapist will utilise Pre-Therapy reflections, as opposed to more orthodox Person-Centred Therapy, in response to those contact functions in which the client is pre-expressive. In reality, however, the borderline between pre-expressive and expressive functioning is not always obvious. Dion van Werde has identified this ambiguous area as 'grey-zone functioning', in which the two modes of functioning are interwoven.

The therapist's interventions should be appropriate to the level of functioning as in Figure 4. In order to work with this mixture, the Pre-

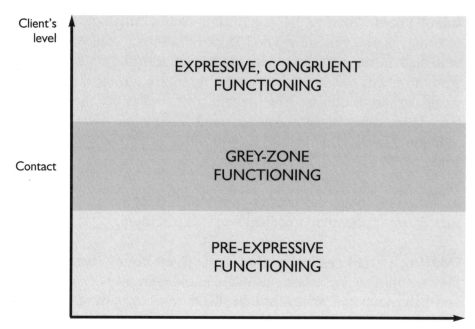

Figure 3 *Client's Level of Functioning*

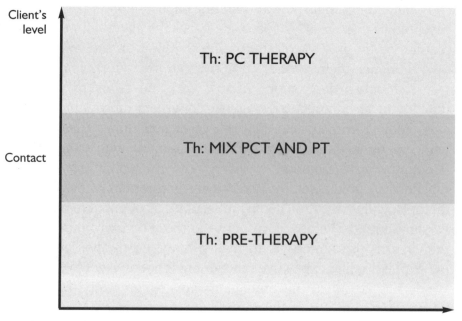

Figure 4 *Therapist's Interventions Matched with Client's Functioning in Practice*

Therapist needs to develop the ability to estimate, and to respond to, the fluctuating level of the client's functioning. Pre-Therapy reflections need to be mastered, in addition to more 'regular' therapeutic interactions, and the therapist should be able to switch from one mode of working to the other in order to match the client's level of functioning. In the case illustration that follows, Dion van Werde demonstrates the reasoning and skills necessary for this task. He is approached in the ward office by a client, Marianne, who has been in hospital for about two weeks. Marianne, for whom psychosis 'is never far away', enters the office slowly. She is staring and speaking in a monotone. Dion is unsure as to whether her initial question expresses psychotic, paranoid content or is based in reality.

Marianne: Are they coming to get me?
Dion (WWR): Are they coming to get me?

[Since Marianne did not react verbally, but kept staring at me with an unchanged body posture, I tried again to bring her into contact with what was actually happening.]

Dion (SR):   You look at me
        (RP):   and ask if they are coming to get you.
Marianne: Are they coming to get me?

[This strengthened my hypothesis that she was in a psychotic state so I reflected what she did with her body as an extra means for anchorage.]

Dion (BR):   Just a second ago you looked up

[and I myself looked at the window in the same way that she had]

        (RP):   and asked 'Are they coming to get me?'
Marianne: I always hear airplanes and things.

[Obviously she was now showing something of her psychotic world. I maintained eye contact and reflected.]

Dion (WWR): I always hear airplanes and things.
Marianne: What do you think? ... I want to know.

[I was not clear what she meant by this question. Was she asking my opinion about the situation, the interaction or about airplanes? Does she mean that these things are going to take her away? In that moment I myself experienced the blend of the two worlds: the reality of our conversation and/or the reality of her paranoid psychotic system. All I felt I could do was to reflect her question and hope that she would clarify to herself and to me.]

Dion (WWR):   You ask me what I think.
Marianne: Are they coming to get me?

[I had a very clear feeling that every word was important but I did not know what she was going through or where these words were leading her. I carefully reflected only what she had given thus making sure not to distract her from her own process.]

Dion (WWR):   Are they coming to get me?
        (RP):   Just a while ago you said 'I always hear airplanes and things.'
        (SR):   Now you are looking at me
        (WWR):   and ask 'Are they coming to get me?'
Marianne: Can I phone home?

[This was a direct question and I gave a congruent answer since I thought that her level of functioning was more congruent and contact reflections were no longer indicated.]

Dion: You already phoned home: what did you agree with them?
Marianne: They are coming at 2pm. It's still one and half hours to wait.

[This was obviously Reality Contact. Her parents were going to pick her up for weekend leave at 2pm and it was indeed only 12:30pm. I continued on a congruent level and made some suggestions.]

Dion: Indeed, so what will you do? Perhaps walk around a bit? Perhaps you could lie down on your bed?
Marianne: Not on my bed, otherwise I think they will come and get me. I'm not sure I would survive.

[Probably my suggestions had induced her to become more psychotic once again, so I returned to Word-for-Word Reflections and tried not to go beyond what she gave me since her anchorage was fragile.]

Dion (WWR): You don't know if you would survive.
    (RP): You say 'I'm not going to lie down, otherwise I think they will come and get me.'
Marianne: I don't know if I will be alive.
Dion (SR): You look at me
    (WWR): and say, 'I don't know if I will be alive.'
    (FR)· Your eyes look sad.
    (BR): You shiver.
Marianne: I don't feel easy at all.

In this last statement Marianne has contacted her feelings. This is Affective Contact. In the interaction which followed, Marianne very adequately talked about her fear of travelling, made a phone call to change the hour of pick-up and empathically understood her mother who tried to reassure her daughter about the pick-up.

(van Werde, 1994, pp126–128)

Therapists working with clients who are diagnosed as psychotic, as having learning disabilities or as both are often presented with messages that appear to be cryptic, or to represent a kind of 'tip of the iceberg' which overlies less accessible material. The intensity with which such messages are expressed, or the degree to which they are repeated, can indicate that such material carries a deep personal significance which may not be immediately apparent to either the therapist or the client. Pre-Therapy does not view such material as regressive but rather as pre-expressive, in that it has the potential to be processed into messages that are both congruent and coherent. At the very least, each of these utterances should be treated as containing meaningful content that may possibly be recovered. This presents a constant challenge to respect the client's attempt to communicate and to make themselves understood to the person they address. They require a grounded, congruent, warm and transparent listener who has the necessary attitude and skills to respond to their unorthodox and often unique forms of communication and behaviour.

Used either as crisis intervention or in daily spontaneous interactions, Pre-Therapy reflections embody the legacy of the person-centred tradition with its vision of a dignified encounter with other human beings, regardless of the nature of their pre-expressive functioning, which may result from psychosis, learning disability, brain damage or dementia.

We will now look at two brief examples of pre-expressive functioning and Pre-Therapy responses to the very concrete messages that it gives. They are some of the many examples of everyday interactions on a psychiatric ward. In both cases there are several possible interpretations of the behaviour and speech, involving some communication that is clearly pre-expressive and some that shows early congruent ('grey-zone') functioning becoming visible. Hence the use of Prouty's Pre-Therapy reflections was indicated. For other illustrations and more extensive case studies involving people with different diagnoses we refer the reader to the existing literature

Example A
It is 2.15 pm. The nurses are in a meeting at their office. Paula knocks on the door and enters. Her knees are bent, her face indicates that she is in pain and she says that she is suffering vaginal bleeding. Earlier, at the same complaint, another nurse had checked her condition and had not found any bleeding. A nurse reports: 'I go with her to her room. Paula sits down on her bed and leaves no room for me, so I take a chair and sit down opposite the other. She sighs.'

Nurse (FR):	You sigh, Paula.
Paula:	Yes, of course! Wouldn't you? All this bleeding! What's going on?
Nurse (WWR):	Bleeding, you say ...
Paula:	Yes! (*and she smiles.*)
Nurse (FR):	You smile ...
Paula:	It is nothing to laugh at, you know!

> Nurse (*partly reacting congruently and partly with a FR*): No, I see that your eyes look sad …
>
> Paula: (*She is silent for a while.*) Yes, and my mother was going to call me at one o'clock and she still hasn't called !!
>
> Nurse (FR, WWR): Your eyes look sad … You expected a phone-call from your mother at one o'clock and she hasn't called yet.
>
> Paula: I have to go to the bathroom now. Will you come back at 3 o'clock?
>
> Nurse (*answering on the same congruent level*): Yes, I'll be here at 3 o'clock.

Paula has opened this encounter with a message that is obviously pre-expressive. The nurse listens to her, trying to make contact and to help her to express herself congruently. As a result, Paula shows that it is hard for her to wait for something that her mother promised to do, but has not yet done. Paula does contact her feelings of impatience, communicates about it and as a consequence, becomes more able to cope with the reality of the situation. This short, informal interaction was sufficient to bring the woman back into contact with herself. The crisis did not escalate and she became able to express congruently what really was on her mind. It appears that waiting for her mother had been very difficult and had been psychotically translated. The nurse provided the right climate and facilitated contact in a non-intrusive way. The patient could again congruently express what was going on. The nurse took her seriously and met her on the same level of concreteness. The patient was able to use her own resources to take the next step by disclosing what was really going on: she felt frustrated since her mother had unexpectedly kept her waiting.

Example B
Everybody is entering the living area and staff are getting ready to start up the weekly ward meeting. Carol, a patient, comes hurrying in and chatters incoherently and continuously. Obviously she is very upset. She communicates experiences that are partly realistic, partly very private:

Carol:	In the cafeteria there is a crucifix in bent wood [*correct*]! There are seances there [*idiosyncratic reality*]! I am permeated by smoke and I do smoke more lately!!
Therapist (WWR):	Carol, you just were in the cafeteria and you saw the crucifix.
(FR):	You look upset.
(WWR):	You talk about seances and smoke.
Carol:	Yes, the closer you get, the more you smoke!
Therapist (FR):	You look concerned.
(RP):	You just came running in from the cafeteria and you are obviously going through a lot just now ...

As a result of the therapist's giving the reflections, the patient's pre-expressive functioning was contained. She found someone to share her turmoil with. This enabled her to put her psychotic concerns in the background and successfully direct her attention to the group meeting. Her delusional thinking returned, however, when the therapists asked each member to say something about how the meeting went. When it was Carol's turn, she said: 'I don't know what it is. The smoke of the cafeteria is already in here as well!' Then, referring to the protocol of the group, the facilitator asked her to focus on how she evaluated the meeting. Carol was then able to say, congruently, that she had been busy with her own thoughts in the main. Paying attention to the contributions of others had been too difficult for her.

Developing Person-Centred Work with Different Target Groups and in Different Settings

Working in a person-centred way with people with impaired functioning is, to many people, an unfamiliar concept. There is a continuous challenge to translate person-centred thought into treatment of specific patient groups by a specific group of caregivers (for example, nurses, psychotherapists, movement therapists) in a specific setting which has its own structural demands, possibilities and limitations. There is a double challenge: to ensure that our efforts are 'person-centred' and also that they are compatible with the demands of the setting. Such challenges have undoubtedly faced other therapists in other areas.

While Person-Centred Therapy has always emphasised the role of the relationship between therapist and client, there has been a continuous development of ideas about the nature of the therapeutic process within such a relationship. As Hart (1970) states, the earliest phase (1940–1950) was characterised by a non-directive approach in which the therapist was expected to be permissive, declining to intervene. The therapist gave unconditional acceptance to the client and techniques were limited to clarifying the content of the client's speech and thoughts. The second phase (1950–1957) has been characterised as 'reflective psychotherapy', with the therapist reflecting underlying feelings and this led into the 'experiential' phase (1957–1980) which began with Rogers' articulation of the necessary and sufficient conditions for therapeutic movement. Attention had now shifted to include the therapist's experience of the relationship, in addition to the feelings of the client. After 1980 the emphasis was less on the techniques of therapy and more on to the basic attitudes of the therapist. Gelso and Carter write:

> According to Rogers, change occurs as a result of an interaction between the therapeutic self (counsellor or the therapist) and the client. There is a strong emphasis on being or existing in a real relationship and on the client experiencing him- or herself within that real relationship. The nature of the therapeutic relationship, however, has been defined by relationship conditions (empathy, positive regard and genuineness) as offered by the therapist.
> (Gelso & Carter, 1985, p212)

Germain Lietaer (1990) summarised his views on the practice of Client-Centred Therapy during the 1970s and 1980s, pointing out how an increasing number of Person-Centred Therapists were allowing themselves a certain degree of process directivity in their work:

The core of the client-centered approach remains constructive personality change and how to facilitate it as a therapist. More attention though has been given to aspects of the therapeutic work which go a little further than 'maintenance reflections' or merely the creation of interpersonal safety ... Most characteristic perhaps – at least in European countries – is the fact that client-centered therapists have shaken off their phobia of directing. The time of the 'don'ts' (Gendlin, 1970) has perhaps passed by forever. Most client-centered therapists no longer feel uneasy when defining their work as an active influencing process in which they try to stimulate the unfolding of the client's experiencing process through task-oriented interventions. As 'process experts' they have found a way to intervene actively without falling into manipulation or authoritarian control. The central principle here is that the experience of the client has to remain the continuous touchstone for what is introduced by the therapist: The therapist must always be receptive and responsive to what his interventions have brought about in the client. We have also witnessed an increased tendency to produce detailed descriptions of interventions specified for different types of client, in different settings and in different processes. Whilst this remains the subject of some debate within the person-centered community, we should remember that Rogers always restricted himself to descriptions of what he saw as the essential features of person-centered work – the 'heart of the matter' – and left it to individual therapists to give it concrete expression. He thus respected the many different individual styles that therapist's brought to their work. We therefore suggest that he would have been comfortable with the current trend, especially strong in Europe, towards an increased differentiation of approaches to meet the needs of specific client groups. Increasingly innovative work is being produced in many different areas.
(Lietaer, 1990, pp33–34)

(Lietaer refers to Prouty's work in his summary of work with people who are severely disturbed.)

Pre-Therapy, which seeks to restore and strengthen psychological contact, can be seen as an example of a specific person-centred approach which serves a broad range of pre-expressive clients. Its overall aim is to work with the ineffective contact functions in order that basic contact with reality and affect, and communication are made possible. This focus fits within the larger person-centred framework, being founded on a strong belief that we are working with human beings, like you and me, involving a conscious effort to separate the person from the disease. Even where functioning has become chaotic or frozen, we seek to help the person regain contact with, and control of, their own life. Although progress is often very modest, it is nonetheless significant. Given the suffering of the people we are working with, progress is seen more in terms of an increased quality of life, involving more time spent ' in contact' and living in 'the here and now' as opposed to traditional psychotherapeutic progression.

People with strengthened contact functions are better equipped to relate to someone who genuinely wishes to help them. When offered the right conditions, it becomes possible for the patient to use again their proactive forces, albeit within their existing limitations. We are trying to enable clients to regain as much control as possible over their own lives in a way that is ultimately, even with these populations, inspired by Rogers' concept of the fully-functioning person.

If we were trying to encapsulate the essence of Pre-Therapy, we might say that we are attempting to guide our clients, and ourselves:

- away from a therapist/client relationship that is characterised by interpretation, control, authoritarianism, structure, product focus, judgementalism;
- away from activity that is characterised by being repetitive, superficial, empty, dull, obligatory;
- away from a level of functioning that is psychotic, inhibited, bizarre, isolated, non-accessible, insecure, covered up, frozen; and
- towards a level of functioning that is experiential, process-oriented, anchored, in-touch, shared, decided, active, creative, varied, concentrated, enjoyed and in process.

The psychotherapist or 'contact facilitator' seeks to contact and to work with the client's tendency to be rooted and operative, to form an alliance with their remaining ability to deal congruently with situations, the areas that still have some strength left. In Pre-Therapy we make contact, accompany, strengthen the anchorage and help the person regain some degree of control over their situation. We need to be realistic, however. Each person is biologically and psychologically unique and some people can make much more progress than others. Some have more courage, others have more strength, others again have suffered more, and received more damage. Some people have others who support them, whereas some have never experienced the feeling of trusting someone, a further group does not want to relinquish their established equilibrium as the suffering it entails appears far less damaging than experiencing (an underlying traumatic) reality. Each process is different. Every quest for strength and health is unique. So is every therapy. Helping somebody is a creative act. The therapist really has to look assiduously for a way to reach this particular fellow person, how to form a relationship and how to strengthen their anchoring. It takes some time and some training to become familiar, and at ease, with this philosophy and this method of working, especially as so many caregivers have been conditioned to take action, to change people. Nobody ever told us that 'being with' a person and giving simple reflections could be so powerful.

It can sometimes be difficult to discern any progress that a client is making. They may, temporarily, suffer increased chaos when old psychological patterns are challenged, when a process of experiencing is restarted and a new sense of equilibrium has to be found. Working on the strengthening of contact functions does not allow us to lose sight of our responsibility for the management of the individual patient. Reality is presented and is worked with, even when this means confronting or restricting the patient. Pre-Therapy does often help to bridge these two interests, as when contact increases, this leads to a decline in symptomatology and, as a result, the patient is better able to adapt to the social environment.

Some caregivers, parents or partners work spontaneously in a way that is similar to Pre-Therapy, but we aim to do it more systematically. This will allow it to be taught, and for its effects to be measured. Most of all, Pre-Therapy gives people the tools to develop a fundamentally empathic and genuine way of taking care of people with pre-expressive features.

Pre-Therapy and Dementia Care

There are two kinds of documented outcome for Pre-Therapy. The most obvious effect is the restoration of the client's contact functions, as they regain access to everyday reality and communication. This is, of course, a very significant result in its own right and it can also lead to a number of secondary gains. Prouty reports the case of a girl with learning disabilities who had acute episodes of aggressive outbursts. As a result of his using Pre-Therapy, she became able to contact her feelings (affective contact) instead of pre-expressively acting them out. The staff could now work with her anger instead of simply cleaning up the mess after her outbursts, as they had in the past. A secondary gain was that the child's mother began to feel secure enough to have her daughter for weekend visits and the staff could allow her to attend workshops during the week. This all, in turn, increased the girl's level of functioning, in that it further consolidated and strengthened the restored contact functions. She regained acceptance from her peer group and restored the confidence of others in her.

A second potential outcome of Pre-Therapy is that the client engages in psychotherapy. In such cases the restoration of contact allows the person to start to explore their affective content and to begin to process the decoded material. Prouty and Kubiak (1988) have reported a crisis intervention which dealt successfully with the problem behaviour of a girl with learning disabilities. This included yelling and screaming, while full of terror and panic, accompanied by a frozen body posture with arms outstretched. Regular sessions of psychotherapy later revealed that this behaviour stemmed from her childhood experience of being punished by her mother, who would attach the hose of the vacuum cleaner to the young girl's arm. After achieving this insight, the girl was able to end ten years of incomprehensible (pre-expressive) behaviour in which she repeatedly caressed and kissed her arm.

In relation to Pre-Therapy and people with dementia, van Werde stipulates another possible outcome. Once impairment is at such a

159

level that restoring functioning becomes unrealistic, it can be seen as the art of 'being with' the someone whose functioning is continuing to decline. It can be considered as an act of 'palliative care'. This resemblance between caring with someone in the later stages of dementia and being with a person who is dying will be illustrated later.

In any event, Pre-Therapy is, by definition, designed to assist contact by the person with impaired functioning. Restoration of contact functions will sometimes be possible, depending on the overall level of functioning. Occasionally, perhaps temporarily, an augmented level may be reached and this type of contact-facilitation is well suited to supporting the 'healthy' or recovered functioning that remains. It may be that, in this sense, the inevitable decline of functioning is slowed down, or temporarily prevented.

Pre-Therapy can also help carers cope with pre-expressive behaviour in a way that is beneficial to the person with dementia. A carer does not need a great deal of experience or skill to be able to use the contact reflections as an inspiration for very concrete responses to the strange and unintelligible behaviour that often accompanies dementia, as is shown in the following brief example. The son in this particular vignette had become familiar with Pre-Therapy and contact reflections at a time when his dementing mother was in significant decline. He is not a psychotherapist and has had no formal training in Pre-Therapy. He uses reflections — in his words — to 'keep the conversation going' by constantly returning to concrete reality. In this interaction he reflects his mother's first sentence (as it was indeed hot in the room) and summarises the rest of her speech ('you are thinking about something else'). The mother then was able to indicate, non-verbally, that she was thirsty. The son's reflections probably enabled the woman to set aside her concern for the hallucinations of her father and pick up the thread of the warm weather and of being thirsty. The son states that he had a very clear impression that his mother used the first part of his remark as a stepping stone to further communication about her thirst.

Mother:	It is warm.
	Do you also see that on the ceiling, that picture?
	My father is visiting me ...

Son (WWR): It is warm and now you are thinking about
something else ...

This son has reported that, without the use of Pre-Therapy reflections, even a ten-minute visit to his mother was a torture, as he easily became lost in pre-expressive communication. By reflecting the concrete, he said, a 'conversation' between the two of them could sometimes last half an hour. He testifies that being with his demented mother became more bearable and opportunities arose to say farewell. Above all, it gave him the feeling of still being able to converse with his mother, which other family members and nurses could no longer do. He felt that the use of reflections made his mother feel herself understood and gave her the opportunity and the necessary time to order and arrange her communicative efforts.

In a more general sense, working with this population is similar to working with people with learning disabilities and psychotic people, as the therapist does not know in advance if recovery of the contact functions is possible, or where the pre-expressive behaviour may lead. We can only be humble and offer our skills and our self as a person in an attempt to make some kind of contact and, depending on the client's pace and capabilities, we will be shown how far this joint venture will take us.

We will conclude by reporting a longer interaction that took place between a different son and his dying mother. The mother had been admitted to a hospital and the family took turns in waiting by her bed. She was suffering a terminal frontal tumour, which produced dementia-like symptoms. The case dramatically illustrates the woman's struggle for congruent communication and experiencing. We see the son trying to make contact by 'being' with her on the same level of concreteness and chaos. Through the use of Pre-Therapy reflections, he is also offering her an invitation to built up her contact level if she is able to do so, if she feels ready and if she wishes to. As a result, we see that, after a pre-expressive struggle, the woman is in the end able to call out the forename and the family name of her son. Given her condition, this was a relatively high-level moment of real contact. For the son, it became a truly sacred moment in what turned out to be their final interaction:

Son	(SR):	Now I'm sitting on this side of the bed.
	(SR):	There is more light here.
	(SR):	I can read better here.
		...
	(SR):	I'm writing a bit.
		...
	(BR):	You hold your hand to your head.
Mother:		I was going to read.
Son	(WWR):	You were going to read.
Mother:		Another paper...
Son	(WWR):	Another paper...
Mother:		'Kellogs?', or what's the name ...
Son (congruent response):		Maalox?
Mother:		Yes.
		What?
Son	(WWR):	What.
Mother:		Whats?
Son	(WWR):	Whats.
Mother:		And which do you have to take than?
Son	(WWR):	And which to take?
	(BR):	You keep your hand to your head.
Mother:		Yes.
		...
Son	(FR):	... and you yawn.
Mother:		Yes. But I have to yawn.
Son	(WWR):	Yes. I have to yawn.
Mother:		Yawn, Yawn.
Son	(WWR):	Yawn.
Mother:		Yes, 'Kellogs'.
Son	(WWR):	'Kellogs'.
Mother:		Yes. The Kellogs book. Yes.
Son	(WWR):	Yes.
	(RP):	I came to sit on this side of the bed ... You were talking ... and your hand was on your head.

Mother:		And that was it.
Son	(WWR):	That was it.
Mother:		That was it, the deliberation.
Son	(WWR):	The deliberation.
		…
		…
Son	(FR):	… and you cough …
Mother:		Yes, a bad cough, … I don't like it a bit.
Son	(WWR):	You don't like it a bit.
	(RP):	You cough and you say: 'I don't like it'.
Mother:		I like it, I don't like it …
		Praying.
Son	(WWR):	Praying …
		I like it, I don't like it …
	(RP):	… and you say 'praying'.
Mother:		Now, I'm happy.
Son	(WWR):	You're happy.
Mother:		Now, I'm happy.
		Where I'm not happy, I am not happy …
		And now I'm happy.
Son	(WWR):	Now you're happy.
Mother:		Yes, that's fine, isn't it …
Son	(WWR):	That's fine.
Mother:		Voilà, that's the way it is. Am I happy, am I happy, am I not happy, am I not happy. That's it.
Son	(WWR):	That's it.
		…
		…
	(RP):	You cough and you said: 'that's it'.
Mother:		And I cough and I cough and I cough.
Son	(WWR):	And you say 'I cough'.
Son	(FR, RP):	A big yawn and you say 'I cough'.
		…
		…
		…
	(SR):	… and you are silent now.

Mother:		Yes.
		...
		...
		Three times, I do good.
Son	(WWR):	Three times, I do good.
Mother:		Mhm mhm ...
		...
		...

(Mother wipes her hand over the sheets.)

Son	(BR):	You wipe with your hand.
Mother:		My hand wipes the little chair.
Son	(WWR):	Your hand wipes the little chair.
Mother:		I wiped the chair.
		Than I wipe loose.
		Than I don't wipe loose ...
Son	(RP):	You wiped the chair.
Mother:		Than I wipe it loose.
Son	(SR):	Your hand is on the pillow.
Mother:		It looks like it, doesn't it ...
Son	(WWR):	It looks like it, doesn't it ...
Mother:		Does somebody finally helps me?
Son	(WWR):	Does somebody finally helps me?
Mother:		Do I get help? Yes, don't I?
Son	(WWR):	You ask if you are getting help.
Mother:		Yes ...
		It is good, isn't it?
Son	(WWR):	You say 'it is good'
Mother:		It is [*unclear* ...]
Son	(WWR):	It is 'of the boys'?
Mother:		Grandiose.
Son (RP, WWR):		I heard 'of the boys' and you say 'grandiose'.
Mother:		That's what I also heard in the beginning, and it isn't true.
Son	(RP):	Grandiose.
Mother:		Why isn't that OK?

Son (WWR):	Why isn't that OK?
Mother:	It is good.
	...
	Yes.
	What is there left to do? What is there left to do?
Son (WWR, BR):	'What is there left to do?' and you hold your hand to your head.
Mother:	What is there still left over than? I want to do something about it though ...
Son (WWR):	I do want to do something about it though.
Mother:	But what?
	...
	Muscles. If all that is good for us ...
	Goodygoodygood ...
Son (WWR, RP):	Goodygoodygood ... What there is still left over...
Mother:	If there still is something left over ... You know what I mean, S.
Son (WWR)	(surprised and very touched): You say my Christian name, 'S'.
Mother:	'S' I say, 'SQ.' (Forename and family name!)
Son (WWR):	'SQ', that's my name!
Mother:	That's your name. That's a beautiful name.
Son:	(S sits closer and caresses the hand of his mother.)
	...
	...
(SR):	And it turned a little bit darker outside ...
Mother:	... and more quiet ...
Son (WWR):	(agreeing and confirming) ... more quiet ...
Mother:	... and more quiet, that pleases me.
Son (WWR):	... and more quiet, that pleases you.
	...
	... quiet ...

Conclusion

We hope that this chapter has indicated some of the potential benefits that Prouty's Pre-Therapy might bring to dementia care. We have described how Pre-Therapy can deal successfully with different types of impaired, or pre-expressive, functioning in the knowledge that the application of Pre-Therapy to dementia care is only just beginning. It will require trained Pre-Therapists and different kinds of contact facilitators to start translating work that has already been developed to this particular field. As can be seen from its application in other areas (for a summary see Prouty *et al*, 1998), Pre-Therapy can be applied in its 'pure' form, or can serve as a source of inspiration for all kinds of daily interaction and even as an overall and organising concept for a therapeutic milieu. A trained contact facilitator will be very well prepared to work with people with dementia, never underestimating the potential for growth in the individual that they are working with. As contact with reality, contact with one's own affective functioning and congruent communication, is the constant focus of attention, the caregiver will be witness, over time, to the declining capabilities of the other. Pre-Therapy then, as a genuine Person-Centred Therapy, will at this stage be brought back to its essence, to the art of existential empathy, to truly 'being with'.

CHAPTER 6

Towards a Person-Centred Culture of Dementia Care?

ALTHOUGH THERE MAY BE grounds for some discussion as to whether Pre-Therapy, with its use of specific 'techniques', is truly 'person-centred' in the Rogerian sense, there is no doubt as to the strength of the conceptual bonds that tie it to the therapeutic tradition initiated by Rogers. Prouty employs constructs that have been fashioned within the person-centred tradition and he has developed both the theory and the practice of Pre-Therapy as an extension — or, in his own words, as an 'evolution' (Prouty, 1994) — of Person-Centred Therapy.

The clarity of Pre-Therapy's relationship with Rogerian thought stands in marked contrast to the ambiguity which surrounds the use of the term 'person-centred' in relation to the 'new culture' of dementia care. The growing use of the term 'person-centred' in relation to dementia care is accompanied by an understanding that owes more to Kitwood than it does to Rogers. This understanding has much in common with the everyday use of phrases outlined at the beginning of Chapter 1, a usage which has spawned related expressions, such as 'student-centred', 'user-centred' or 'patient focused' — terms which, although indirectly betraying some of the characteristics of Rogerian thought, also carry significant differences from it.

So what is meant by term 'person-centred' when it is used in relation to dementia care? Usage often implies that it conveys how the 'person' is being held uppermost in the thoughts of those who are planning and delivering care. This prompts a further question: the 'person' as opposed to what? What was uppermost in carers' minds before person-centred care arrived on the scene? The answer that first comes to mind is that in the 'old culture' of dementia care the centre stage of carers' concerns was occupied by, in varying combinations, the disease, the needs of the caring organisation or, more recently, the needs of family carers. The presence of 'someone on the inside' of the dementia — an experiencing, sentient being 'just like me' — was somehow being overlooked. Kitwood expanded on the centrality of this concern with the person by introducing the social–psychological concept of 'personhood' to dementia care, but it is doubtful, at least at this stage, whether this idea has permeated as widely as his interpretation of 'person-centredness'.

Thus person-centred dementia care can be seen as something of an antidote, a corrective measure, for the deformations of dementia care that preceded its arrival during the shift that Kitwood christened the 'New Culture of Dementia Care'. It represents an attempt to refocus on the real issue for dementia care — the person and the quality of their life — and as such its adherents do carry similarities with those in other fields of human activity who aspire to be 'student-centred', 'user-centred' or 'patient focused'. These phrases, always employed in relation to the servicing of some human need or desire, are also indicative of a will to refocus on the fundamental purpose, the primary goal, of the organisation or of the collective effort. They carry an acknowledgement that other factors and needs, particularly the needs of the organisation itself or of individuals and interest groups within the organisation, can obscure, or deflect from, such primary goals.

In such contexts, 'person-centred' has come to indicate projects which attempt to replicate, in their own field, the same type of achievements that Rogers made in psychotherapy. The use of the same expression does not represent a theoretical or conceptual link to Rogers so much as it signals a similarity to his motivations and to the objectives of his project: to correct those deformations in theory and practice which came to obscure (and thereby prevent the achievement of) psychotherapy's primary goals. It is also worth noting that such goals tend to be generally understood in terms of the delivery of some service to individuals, as opposed to the fulfilment of some collective need, an understanding that resonates with Rogers' historical position within the tradition of Protestant individualism (Prouty, 1994, p3).

This claim, that a person-centred approach emerged primarily as a corrective response to the deformations which had previously characterised virtually the entire field of dementia care, is supported by the fact that Kitwood's earliest work consisted largely of attacks on the contemporary theory (the standard paradigm) and practice (the 'Malignant Social Psychology') of dementia care.

Recent Developments in British Dementia Care: The Flowering of a Person-Centred Culture?

The diversity and innovation which have characterised the renaissance of dementia care in Britain are illustrated by the breadth of innovation and variety of material contained in the bi-monthly *Journal of Dementia Care*. A well-read practitioner of dementia care in the 1980s would have difficulty believing that the following decade would open such possibilities for advance in their field. Where once we were limited to the use of Reality Orientation, we now have a wide and ever-expanding repertoire of approaches at our disposal.

Elements of person-centred thought can be traced throughout this new culture, even if many of the advances consist largely of a rectification of the deficits of the old culture of care. Indeed, what we have witnessed can be seen as a continuation of the breaking down of the barriers between dementia care and other areas of mental health care, barriers that were initially breached by Stokes and Goudie's Resolution Therapy. From aromatherapy to the various creative therapies, from behaviour modification to psychotherapy, practitioners of dementia care are increasingly adventurous and confident in looking to adapt and apply skills and knowledge that have their roots in other areas of mental health.

To what extent can these developments be described as 'person-centred' in its original, Rogerian, sense? Towards the end of Chapter 1 were listed eight features of 'person-centredness' and we began to explore their relevance to the field of dementia care. It seems appropriate to conclude by returning to those features and asking how far current practice has moved to embrace them.

A respect for the Subjective Experiences,
Perceptions and 'Inner' World of the Individual

In order to appreciate another person's frame of reference, we must first learn to listen. There are clear signs of a growing awareness of the importance of actually listening to people with dementia, continuing a strand that has run through the work of Feil, Goudie and Stokes, and Kitwood. More recently, it has formed the subject of an optimistic and inspiring book by Malcolm Goldsmith. His work on communication with people with dementia (Goldsmith, 1996a) is based on a recognition of the need for empathic concern: 'We have to be willing to try and enter their "world", with all its alternative boundaries and conventions, rather than expect them to respond to ours' (Goldsmith, 1996b, p25). Goldsmith's optimistic response to the challenge of involving people with dementia in the planning of the provision of services is shared by Keady *et al*'s (1995) report on interviews undertaken with people who have relatively mild cognitive impairment.

The many hours that John Killick has spent listening to people with dementia, in his work as writer in residence in units for people with dementia, have led him to echo Cheston's observations (Cheston, 1996) when he states that: 'It seems to me that the language used by people with dementia is a metaphorical one' (Killick, 1994, p17). Killick also shares Feil's view of the poetic use of language in dementia and has used his conversations with people with dementia to produce a series of poems (Killick, 1997). His poetry reveals how the apparently disjointed communication of people with dementia often betrays a far deeper understanding and appreciation of their experience than we realise.

The extent to which we, with our memories intact and our experience relatively integrated, can hope to get inside the experience of dementia is open to debate. We saw in Chapter 4 that Tom Kitwood suggested that there are seven 'access routes' by which we: 'can gain insight into the subjective world of dementia' (Kitwood, 1997a, pp73–79). These 'routes', which include role-play and reading accounts by people who have dementia, will undoubtedly help us gain some insight into the general experience of dementia, but achieving empathy with people who have a significant degree of cognitive impairment remains problematic. We may be able to empathise with, and respond empathically to, the emotions that an individual's subjective experiences provoke, but we also have to admit there are significant obstacles to our gaining a true insight into their frame of reference. Chief amongst such obstacles are the limitations of our own past experience. I cannot, for example, fully appreciate what it is like to be unable to remember what happened 30 seconds ago. When such limitations are combined with either the lack of communication or with the problems we have understanding the communication of people with dementia, we may well be forced to admit that the kind of empathy that is achievable is more in line with that Prouty describes as characteristic of the relationship with people who are deep in psychoses: 'The therapist does not know the client's frame of reference. The empathy is for the client's effort at developing coherent experience and expression' (Prouty, 1994, p49).

A Non-Judgemental Acceptance of the Unique Qualities of Each Individual
It may appear strange to the reader who is new to dementia care to suggest that a widespread appreciation of the need to actually listen to people with dementia is a relatively recent development. The same can be said of the growing recognition of the need for individualised care, grounded both in a knowledge of the past history of the person with dementia and in some appreciation of their frame of reference. These themes preoccupied many of the case studies in the 'Person-Centred Care' series which the *Journal of Dementia Care* ran over 13 issues from 1995 to 1997. This series was heavy with an (unstated) awareness of our historic failing to acknowledge the individuality of people with dementia, to take their views into account or to even attempt to understand their experience.

It is likely that this failing was a price that was unwittingly paid for the manner in which the public were encouraged — by an earlier generation of health professionals — to understand that people with dementia should not be held morally responsible, or blamed, for the results of their cognitive deficits. The widespread explanation that 'it's not really them, its their illness' encouraged a new form of judgementalism, in which the behaviour and speech of people with dementia were understood purely in terms of their neuropathology.

Kitwood's plea for us to 'Discover the Person, not the Disease' (Kitwood, 1993a) invited us to move beyond this position.

An Emphasis on Seeing the Person 'as a Whole'
We need to acknowledge that the breadth and variety of innovation in the field of dementia care are indicative of an increasingly holistic approach. A number of articles indicate how issues such as the sexuality (see, for example, Archibald, 1994) and the spirituality (for example, Barnett, 1995) of people with dementia are being addressed. We are also seeing a growth in the diversity of creative and sensory therapies, many of which have their origins in the care of people with learning disabilities. Such developments show how the belief that the person with dementia remains a 'person' above all else is becoming a basic tenet in the minds of many involved with dementia care.

A Positive View of Human Nature and its Tendency to Fulfil its Potential
Rogers' reflections on his own ageing (Rogers, 1980, pp70–95; 1987) seem to imply that he saw getting older as being very much a continuation, or an expansion, of his earlier development, although he does point out that in the decade between his 65th and 75th birthdays he developed a tendency to take far more risks of various kinds than he was ever inclined to before. There is little evidence that he saw old age as a distinct developmental stage or as involving preparation for death (indeed, these writings are rather more preoccupied with conjectures about the possibility of life after death). We are probably safe, therefore, in assuming that Rogers believed in the capacity of human nature to continue moving towards fulfilling its potential.

While reframing dementia as a positive developmental experience is generally regarded as an act of insensitive folly, the more holistic appreciation of the person with dementia has at least drawn attention to those (non-cognitive) aspects of being human in which individuals might continue to grow.

An Elevation of the Importance Attached to Feelings and Emotions
Tom Kitwood's work on 'relative well-being' in dementia was initially put forward as a list of twelve indicators of well-being, each of which

related to affect (Kitwood & Bredin, 1992a). He stressed the importance of both 'positive' and 'negative' emotions, as the latter are an integral part of everyday life which accompany the losses experienced in dementia and in old age. Dementia Care Mapping, which involves observers spending many hours considering the emotional well-being of people with dementia, has made a very significant practical contribution to the spreading of this concern.

The growing interest in the potential relationship between various forms of psychotherapy and dementia is also indicative of a general desire to enhance our abilities to assist with the emotional effects of dementia. The formation of 'Psychotherapy and Dementia' interest groups and the appearance of publications (for example, Hausman, 1992; Sinason, 1992) are signs that work in this area is gathering momentum.

An Accent on the Importance of Interpersonal Relationships
This is the area in which there remains much potential for valuable work to be done. The experience of Spring Mount has shown the degree to which individuals with dementia can form social relationships as part of a group and Kitwood stressed the key role that relationships, as an inherent part of preserving personhood, play in maintaining well-being.

As was mentioned in Chapter 1, however, little work has been done to identify any impact that dementia might have on our capacity to form mutually satisfying human relationships. There is a mass of anecdotal evidence to suggest that the formation of relationships in dementia is remarkably free of cognitive restraints. Given that our most profound relationships are formed in earliest infancy, well before we develop a capacity to use or understand language, this should not, perhaps, surprise us. Paula Crimmens, a drama therapist who has drawn on the ideas of the American anthropologist Stanley Kellerman, paid particular attention to the development of non-verbal communication skills with which carers will need to be equipped in order to build therapeutic relationships with people with dementia (Crimmens, 1995).

An Acknowledgement of the Value of Authenticity in Such Relationships
Kitwood laid great emphasis on the way in which a carer's need to maintain a 'professional distance' can hinder the growth of therapeutic

relationships with people with dementia (Kitwood, 1997a, pp118–132). His concerns echo Bell and McGregor's efforts to prevent the appearance of an 'us and them' relationship emerging between staff and residents at Spring Mount. Such relationships are, of course, the norm in dementia care and there is at least some degree of recognition that they will not be easy to shift. Kitwood argued that professional distance serves to protect us from painful insight into our own deficiencies (Kitwood & Bredin, 1992a) and this in turn implies that most care staff will require a far deeper level of psychological and developmental support than they currently receive. His suggestion that caregivers' development requires either psychotherapy or meditation (Kitwood, 1997, p130–132) may currently be far from the agenda of most organisations providing care, although the Bradford Group is offering training in 'The Depth Psychology of Dementia Care' and this training agenda is also being taken forward by others (for example, Loveday, 1998).

At a more basic level, it would be wrong to assume that simple, factual, honesty is universally accepted as a precondition to developing a helping relationship with someone with dementia. Caregivers continue to be tempted to use subtle deceptions, exploiting their superior factual understanding of the situation to gain the results they require. One article published as part of the *Journal of Dementia Care's* 'Person-Centred Care' series described how a hospitalised man with dementia had his belief that he was in a top-class hotel constantly reinforced and was even persuaded to take tranquillising medication by being: 'told that it had been sent specially for him by the management' (Wallace, 1996).

A Non-Directive Approach

When every carer, in every situation, is endeavouring to maximise the degree of control and choice available to the person with dementia, then we shall have achieved a non-directive approach. We may have a considerable way to go before realising this aspiration, but the general trend is moving in this direction and increasing skills in communicating with, and establishing the choices of, people with dementia will open up more possibilities.

With regard to residential care, physical and organisational design factors can have a significant impact on the autonomy that individuals can exercise. A visitor to Spring Mount, for example, cannot but be impressed by its large and interesting grounds. In Britain, the Domus Project (Lindesay *et al*, 1991; Murphy *et al*, 1994) has paid particular attention to the need for people with dementia to retain a sense of agency, which is also a feature of the growth in group home living in Sweden (Keady & Lundh, 1997).

To be non-directive in our communication with people with dementia poses a far greater challenge and, while progress may have been made in persuading caregivers to be less directive, it appears that only Pre-Therapy can lay claim to being truly non-directive. Given that it took Rogers and supporters of the Person-Centred Therapy many years of concerted effort to minimise traces of directive elements in their own approach, it would only be realistic to suggest that those of us who are involved with dementia care, whose culture is steeped in a tradition of control, still have enormous room for progress in this regard.

There is now a widespread acknowledgement that there has been a significant advance in dementia care in Britain, an advance which began in the late 1980s and which has continued, with increased momentum, ever since. While there is much room for debate about the causes of this advance — and about the degree to which it has permeated into the actual lives of real people with dementia — it seems clear that its beginning was marked by the breaching of the conceptual 'Berlin Wall' that had grown up between 'organic' and 'functional' mental illnesses and between their treatments. Once this divide had been breached, and once those on the 'organic' side began to appreciate that there was much they could learn from ideas and approaches developed outside their own field, some degree of person-centred influence was assured. But why has so much of the 'new culture' of dementia care defined itself as being person-centred, even when there has been an almost complete lack of contact between those working in dementia care and those working within the person-centred tradition? The answer lies, perhaps, in the fact that those pioneers who have formed the subject of this book were both well aware of, and heavily influenced by, Rogers and by the person-centred tradition. While the thought of each may also have been shaped by numerous other influences, it was the person-centred aspects of their approaches which spoke most clearly to the frustrated aspirations of carers to begin to meet the emotional needs of people with dementia. Despite the numerous, powerful forces which would seek to persuade us otherwise, most people in our society still place great value on relationships which involve a depth of contact, honesty, mutuality and regard. Despite the numerous and powerful obstacles which can be created by cognitive impairment, an increasing number now aspire to such relationships with people who have dementia.

References

Archibald C, *Sexuality and Dementia: A Guide,* Dementia Services Development Centre, Stirling, 1994.

Barnett E, 'Broadening our Approach to Spirituality', Kitwood T & Benson S (eds), *The New Culture of Dementia Care,* pp40–43, Hawker Publications, London, 1995.

Bell J & McGregor I, 'Breaking Free from Myths that Restrain us', *Journal of Dementia Care* 2(4), pp14–15, 1994.

Bell J & McGregor I, 'A Challenge to Stage Theories of Dementia', Kitwood T & Benson S (eds), *The New Culture of Dementia Care,* pp12–14, Hawker Publications, London, 1995.

Bleathman C & Morton I, 'Validation Therapy: Extracts from Groups with Dementia Sufferers', *Journal of Advanced Nursing* 17, pp658–666, 1992.

Bleathman C & Morton I, 'Psychological Treatments', Burns A & Levy R (eds), *Dementia,* pp553–64, Chapman & Hall, London, 1994.

Bower GH, 'Mood and Memory', *American Psychologist* 3b, pp129–148, 1981.

Brazier D, 'The Necessary Condition is Love: Going Beyond Self in the Person-Centred Approach', Brazier D (ed), *Beyond Carl Rogers: Towards a Psychotherapy for the 21st Century,* pp72–91, Constable, London, 1993.

Bredin K, Kitwood T & Wattis J, 'Decline in Quality of Life for Patients with Severe Dementia Following a Ward Merger', *International Journal of Geriatric Psychiatry* 10(11), pp967–973, 1995.

Butler RN, 'The Life Review: An Interpretation of Reminiscence in the Aged', *Psychiatry* 26, pp65–76, 1963.

Cheston R, 'Stories and Metaphors: Talking About the Past in a Psychotherapy Group for People with Dementia', *Ageing and Society* 16, pp579–602, 1996.

Crimmens P, 'Beyond Words: To the Core of Human Need for Contact', *Journal of Dementia Care* 3(6), pp12–14, 1995.

De Klerk Rubin V, 'How Validation is Misunderstood', *Journal of Dementia Care* 2(2), pp14–16, 1994.

Erikson E, *Childhood and Society*, Norton, New York, 1950.

Evans RI, *Carl Rogers: The Man and His Ideas*, EP Dutton, New York, 1975.

Feil N, 'Group Therapy in a Home for the Aged', *The Gerontologist* 7(3), pp192–195, 1967.

Feil N, 'A New Approach to Group Therapy with Senile Psychotic Aged', unpublished paper presented at the 25th Annual Meeting of the Gerontological Society, 1972a.

Feil N, 'Proposal for Research Project for Aged Mentally Impaired Senile', unpublished, 1972b.

Feil N, 'Study Guide for video "Looking for Yesterday"', Feil Productions, Cleveland, 1978.

Feil N, *V/F Validation: The Feil Method*, 1st edn, Feil Productions, Cleveland, 1982.

Feil N, *V/F Validation: The Feil Method*, rev. 2nd edn, Feil Productions, Cleveland, 1992a.

Feil N, 'Validation Therapy with Late-Onset Dementia Populations', Jones GMM & Miesen BML (eds), *Care-Giving in Dementia: Research and Applications*, pp199–218, Routledge, London, 1992b.

Feil N, *The Validation Breakthrough*, Health Professions Press, Cleveland, 1993.

Fox L, 'Mapping the Advance of the New Culture of Dementia Care', Kitwood T & Bensen S (eds), *The New Culture of Dementia Care*, pp70–74, Hawker Publications, London, 1995.

Fraser C, 'Social Psychology', Gregory RL (ed), *The Oxford Companion to the Mind*, pp721–723, Oxford University Press, Oxford, 1987.

Gelso CJ & Carter JA, 'The relationship in counseling and psychotherapy: Components, consequences, and theoretical antecedents', *The Counseling Psychologist* 13, pp155–243, 1985.

Gendlin ET, 'A Theory of Personality Change', Hart JT & Tomlinson TM (eds), *New Directions in Client-Centered Therapy*, pp129–173, Houghton Mifflin, Boston, 1970.

Godden DR & Baddeley AD, 'Context-Dependent Memory in Two Natural Environments: On Land and Underwater', *British Journal of Psychology* 66, pp325–331, 1975.

Goldsmith M, *Hearing the Voice of People with Dementia*, Jessica Kingsley, London, 1996a.

Goldsmith M, 'Slow Down and Listen to Their Voice', *Journal of Dementia Care* 4(4), pp24–25, 1996b.

Goudie F & Stokes G, 'Understanding Confusion', *Nursing Times* 85(39), pp35–37, 1989.

Gubrium JR & Lynott RJ, 'Alzheimer's Disease as Biographical Work', Peterson WA & Quadagno J (eds), *Social Bonds in Later Life*, Sage, Beverly Hills, 1985.

Hart JT, 'The Development of Client-Centered Therapy', Hart JT & Tomlinson TM (eds), *New Directions in Client-Centered Therapy*, pp3–22, Houghton Mifflin, Boston, 1970.

Hausman C, 'Dynamic Psychotherapy with Elderly Demented Patients', Jones GMM & Miesen BML (eds), *Care-Giving in Dementia: Research and Applications*, pp181–198, Routledge, London, 1992.

Holden UP & Woods RT, *Reality Orientation: Psychological Approaches to the 'Confused' Elderly,* Churchill Livingstone, Edinburgh, 1982.

Hughes CP, Berg L, Danziger WL, Coben LA & Martin RL, 'A New Clinical Scale for the Staging of Dementia', *British Journal of Psychiatry* 140, pp566–572, 1982.

Jones M, *The Therapeutic Community: A New Treatment Method in Psychiatry*, Basic Books, New York, 1953.

Keady J & Lundh U, 'Living Together: Group Homes in Sweden', *Journal of Dementia Care* 5(3), pp26–28, 1997.

Keady J, Nolan M & Gilliard J, 'Listen to the Voices of Experience', *Journal of Dementia Care* 3(3), pp15–16, 1995.

Killick J, 'There's So Much to Hear When You Stop and Listen to Individual Voices', *Journal of Dementia Care* 2(5), pp16–17, 1994.

Killick J, *You are Words*, Hawker Publications, London, 1997.

Kirschenbaum H, *On Becoming Carl Rogers*, Delta, New York, 1980.

Kitwood T, 'Dementia and its Pathology: in Brain, Mind or Society?', *Free Associations* 8, pp81–93, 1987a.

Kitwood T, 'Explaining Senile Dementia: the Limits of Neuropathological Research', *Free Associations* 10, pp117–140, 1987b.

Kitwood T, 'Brain, Mind and Dementia: With Particular Reference to Alzheimer's Disease', *Ageing and Society* 9, pp1–15, 1989.

Kitwood T, 'The Dialectics of Dementia: With Particular Reference to Alzheimer's Disease', *Ageing and Society* 10(2), pp177–196, 1990a.

Kitwood T, 'Understanding Senile Dementia: A Psychobiolographical Approach', *Free Associations* 19, pp60–76, 1990b.

Kitwood T, 'Psychotherapy and Dementia', *Psychotherapy Section Newsletter* 8, pp40–56, 1990c.

Kitwood T, 'How Valid is Validation Therapy?', *Geriatric Medicine* 22(3), p23, 1992.

Kitwood T, 'Discover the Person not the Disease', *Journal of Dementia Care* 1(1), pp16–17, 1993a.

Kitwood T, 'Towards a Theory of Dementia Care: The Interpersonal Process', *Ageing and Society* 13(1), pp51–67, 1993b.

Kitwood T, 'Charting the Course of Quality Care', *Journal of Dementia Care* 2(3), pp22–23, 1994.

Kitwood T, 'Cultures of Care: Tradition and Change', Kitwood T & Benson S (eds), *The New Culture of Dementia Care*, pp7–11, Hawker Publications, London, 1995.

Kitwood T, *Dementia Reconsidered: The Person Comes First*, Open University Press, Buckingham, 1997a.

Kitwood T, 'The concept of personhood and its relevance for a new culture of dementia care', Miesen BML & Jones GMM (eds), *Care-Giving in Dementia: Research and Applications, Volume 2*, Routledge, London, 1997b.

Kitwood T & Bredin K, 'Towards a Theory of Dementia Care: Personhood and Well-Being', *Ageing and Society* 12(3), pp269–287, 1992a.

Kitwood T & Bredin K, *Person to Person: A Guide to the Care of Those with Failing Mental Powers*, Gale Centre Publications, Loughton, 1992b.

Laing RD, *The Divided Self*, Tavistock, London, 1960.

Lietaer G, 'The client-centered approach after the Wisconsin Project: A personal view on its evolution', Lietaer G, Rombauts J & Van Balen R (eds), *Client-Centered and Experiential Psychotherapy in the Nineties*, Universitaire Pers, Louvain, 1990.

Lindesay J, Briggs K, Lawes M, Macdonald A & Herzberg J, 'The Domus Philosophy: A Comparative Evaluation of a New Approach to Residential Care for the Demented Elderly', *International Journal of Geriatric Psychiatry* 6, pp727–736, 1991.

Loveday B, 'Training to Promote Person-Centered Care', *Journal of Dementia Care* 6(2), pp22–24, 1998.

Makin A, 'The Social Model of Disability', *Journal of the British Association for Counselling* 6(4), p274, 1995.

McGregor I & Bell J, 'Beyond the Mask of Conventional Manners', *Journal of Dementia Care* 2(6), pp20–21, 1994b.

Mearns D & Thorne B, *Person-Centred Counselling in Action*, Sage, London, 1988.

Morton I, 'Beyond Validation', Normal IJ & Redfern SJ (eds), *Mental Health Care for Elderly People,* pp371–391, Churchill Livingstone, Edinburgh, 1997.

Morton I & Bleathman C, 'Reality Orientation: Does it Matter Whether it's Tuesday or Friday?', *Nursing Times* 84(6), pp25–27, 1988.

Murphy E, Lindesay J & Dean R, *The Domus Project: Long Term Care for Older People with Dementia,* The Sainsbury Centre, London, 1994.

O'Dwyer M & Orrell MW, 'Stress, Ageing and Dementia', *International Review of Psychiatry* 6, pp73–83, 1994.

Oliver M, *Social Work with Disabled People,* Macmillan, London, 1983.

Packer T, Bidder V, Lewis J & Maller L, 'Shining a Light of Simple, Crucial Details', *Journal of Dementia Care* 4(6), pp22–23, 1996.

Pattie AH & Gilleard CJ, *Manual of the Clifton Assessment Procedures for the Elderly (CAPE),* Hodder & Stoughton Educational, Sevenoaks, 1979.

Perrin T, 'Occupational Need in Dementia: A Descriptive Study', *Journal of Advanced Nursing* 25, pp934–941, 1997.

Peters H, *Psychotherapie bij geestelijk gehandicapten,* Lisse, Swets & Zeitlinger, Amsterdam, 1992.

Pörtner M, 'Ernstnehmen, Zutrauen, Verstehen. Personzentrierte Haltung im Umgang mit geistig behinderten und pflegebedürftigen Menschen', Prouty G, van Werde D & Pörtner M (eds), *Prä-Therapie,* pp130–141, Klett-Cotta, Stuttgart, 1996.

Prouty G, 'Pre-Therapy — a method of treating pre-expressive psychotic and retarded patients', *Psychotherapy: Theory, Research and Practice,* 13(3), pp290–295, 1976.

Prouty G, *Theoretical Evolutions in Person-Centered/Experiential Therapy: Applications to Schizophrenic and Retarded Psychoses,* Praeger, Westport, 1994.

Prouty G & Kubiak MA, 'Pre-Therapy Applied to Crisis Intervention with a Schizophrenic Retardate', *Psychiatric Aspects of Mental Retardation Reviews* 7(10), pp62–68, 1988.

Prouty G, van Werde D & Pörtner M, *Prä-Therapie,* Klett-Cotta, Stuttgart, 1998.

Roach M, *Another Name for Madness,* Houghton Mifflin, Boston, 1985.

Robertson C, Warrington J & Eagles JM, 'Relocation Mortality in Dementia: The Effects of a New Hospital', *International Journal of Geriatric Psychiatry* 9, pp521–525, 1993.

Rogers CR, *Client-Centered Therapy,* Constable, London, 1951.

Rogers CR, 'A Note on "The Nature of Man"', *Journal of Counselling Psychology* 4(3), pp199–203, 1957a.

Rogers CR, 'The Necessary and Sufficient Conditions of Therapeutic Personality Change', *Journal of Consulting Psychology* 21(2), pp95–103, 1957b.

Rogers CR, 'The Characteristics of a Helping Relationship', *Personnel and Guidance Journal* 37, pp6–16, 1958.

Rogers CR, 'A Theory of Therapy, Personality and Interpersonal Relationships, as Developed in the Client-Centered Framework', Kock S (ed), *Psychology: A Study of a Science, Vol. 3, Formulations of the Person and the Social Context,* pp184–256, McGraw-Hill, New York, 1959.

Rogers CR, *On Becoming a Person,* Houghton Mifflin, Boston, 1961.

Rogers CR, *A Way of Being,* Houghton Mifflin, Boston, 1980.

Rogers CR, 'On Reaching 85', *Person-Centered Review* 2(2), pp150–152, 1987.

Scrutton S, *Counselling Older People,* Edward Arnold, London, 1989.

Sinason V, *Mental Handicap and the Human Condition,* Free Association Books, London, 1992.

Stokes G & Goudie F, 'Counselling Confused Elderly People', Stokes G & Goudie F (eds), *Working with Dementia,* pp181–90, Winslow Press/Speechmark Publishing, Bicester, 1990.

Taulbee LR & Folsom JC, 'Reality Orientation for Geriatric Patients', *Hospital and Community Psychiatry* 17, pp133–135, 1966.

Thorne B, *Carl Rogers,* Sage, London, 1992.

Van Amelsvoort Jones GM, 'Validation Therapy, a Companion to Reality Orientation', *The Canadian Nurse* 81(3), pp20–23, 1985.

Van Werde D, 'Dealing with the possibility of psychotic content in a seemingly congruent communication', Mearns D (ed), *Developing Person Centred Counselling,* pp125–128, Sage, London, 1994.

Wallace D, 'Perfect Manners Demand a First Class Service', *Journal of Dementia Care* 4(4), pp18–19, 1996.

Wolfensberger W, 'Social Role Valorization: a Proposed New Term for the Principle of Normalization', *Mental Retardation* 21, pp234–239, 1983.

Woods RT, 'What Can be Learned from Studies on Reality Orientation?', Jones GMM & Miesen BML (eds), *Care-Giving Dementia: Research and Applications,* pp121–136, Routledge, London, 1992.

Woods RT, 'The Beginnings of a New Culture in Care', Kitwood T & Benson S (eds), *The New Culture of Dementia Care,* pp19–23, Hawker Publications, London, 1995.

Index

INDEX